Cochlear Implant Patient Assessment

Evaluation of Candidacy, Performance, and Outcomes

Core Clinical Concepts in Audiology

Series Editor
Brad Stach, PhD

Basic Audiometry
Editors
James W. Hall III & Virginia Ramachandran

Pure-Tone Audiometry and Masking by Maureen Valente, PhD
Basic Audiometry Learning Manual by Mark DeRuiter, PhD, and Virginia Ramachandran, AuD
Speech Audiometry by Gary D. Lawson, PhD, and Mary E. Peterson, PhD

Electrodiagnostic Audiology
Editors
James W. Hall III & Virginia Ramachandran

Objective Assessment of Hearing by James W. Hall III, PhD, and De Wet Swanepoel, PhD
Otoacoustic Emissions: Principles, Procedures, and Protocols by Sumitrajit Dhar
and James W. Hall III

Cochlear Implants
Editors
Terry Zwolan & Jace Wolfe

Programming Cochlear Implants by Jace Wolfe, PhD, and Erin C. Schafer, PhD
Objective Measures in Cochlear Implants by Michelle L. Hughes, PhD, CCC-A
*Cochlear Implant Patient Assessment: Evaluation of Candidacy,
Performance, and Outcomes* by René H. Gifford, PhD

Vestibular Assessment
Editors
Ken Bouchard & Virginia Ramachandran

Vestibular Learning Manual by Bre L. Myers, AuD
ENG/VNG by Devin L. McCaslin

Cochlear Implant Patient Assessment

Evaluation of Candidacy, Performance, and Outcomes

René H. Gifford, PhD
Vanderbilt University
Assistant Professor, Department of Hearing and Speech Sciences
Director, Cochlear Implant Program, and Associate Director, Pediatric Audiology,
Vanderbilt Bill Wilkerson Center

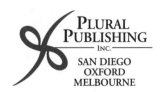

PLURAL
PUBLISHING
INC.
SAN DIEGO
OXFORD
MELBOURNE

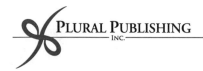

5521 Ruffin Road
San Diego, CA 92123

e-mail: info@pluralpublishing.com
Web site: http://www.pluralpublishing.com

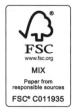

Typeset in 11/13 Palatino by Flanagan's Publishing Services, Inc.
Printed in the United States of America by McNaughton & Gunn

For permission to use material from this text, contact us by
Telephone: (866) 758-7251
Fax: (888) 758-7255
e-mail: permissions@pluralpublishing.com

Every attempt has been made to contact the copyright holders for material originally printed in another source. If any have been inadvertently overlooked, the publishers will gladly make the necessary arrangements at the first opportunity.

Author photo on the back cover copyright © Melanie G Photography, Mt. Juliet, TN.

Library of Congress Cataloging-in-Publication Data

Gifford, Rene H.
  Cochlear implant patient assessment : evaluation of candidacy, performance, and outcomes / Rene H. Gifford.
       p. ; cm.
  Includes bibliographical references and index.
  ISBN-13: 978-1-59756-446-5 (alk. paper)
  ISBN-10: 1-59756-446-X (alk. paper)
  I. Title.
  [DNLM: 1. Cochlear Implants. 2. Cochlear Implantation. 3. Hearing Impaired Persons—rehabilitation. 4. Hearing Loss—rehabilitation. 5. Outcome and Process Assessment (Health Care)—methods. 6. Patient Selection. WV 274]
  LC Classification not assigned
  617.8'9—dc23
                    2012043311

Contents

Preface

Coursework included in the education of student clinicians and educators in the fields of audiology, speech-language pathology, and deaf education tends to focus considerable attention on the history and evolution of cochlear implants including iterations in implant design, signal processing, and recipient outcomes. This information is infinitely valuable and necessary to understand cochlear implants and to ultimately apply that knowledge to the patient and student. What tends to be overlooked in academic instruction, however, is the applied knowledge base required for everyday clinical practice—something that cannot generally be imparted solely from clinical and educational practicum. Clinicians from around the country have phoned and emailed with questions regarding candidate selection, preoperative evaluation protocol, counseling, and postoperative assessment. Questions range from recommending implantation for patients who may not fit the traditional implant candidate profile to sound-field calibration for pre- and post-implant testing to recommendations for additional assessments that may yield diagnostic information not currently provided by the standard battery. Over the past several years of intercepting such questions and interest from students and practicing clinicians, it has become obvious that either this information is not being covered in current academic education or more likely that no such "instructional manual" exists to aid the clinical education for the student clinician or even the professional education of the seasoned clinician. Given that the numbers of adult and pediatric implant recipients continue to increase, more clinicians will be expected to gain and maintain a level of experience surrounding the clinical management of this special population. This book can serve as a guidebook delivering clinically relevant information to audiologists, speech-language pathologists, and deaf educators regarding the assessment tools and therapeutic intervention that are critical during the pre- and post-implant periods.

Acknowledgments

There are a number of individuals to whom I must express my sincerest gratitude for their contributions and assistance in completing this book. First, I would like to individually thank my contributors. Emily Lund, MS, CCC-SLP, graciously offered her writing and clinical expertise in childhood hearing loss and speech-language pathology for Chapters 4 and 8. She has been a delightful student and colleague and I greatly value her opinion and knowledge. I must also thank Dr. Melanie Schuele for not only allowing her PhD student, Emily, to prepare these chapters, but also for graciously offering her expertise in proofreading the chapters.

My Chapter 1 coauthors—Deb Arthur, Pat Macy, and Cedric Navarro—are truly amazing experts on all matters of implant regulation. They have taught me so much more than I could ever imagine about a dry, yet dramatically important topic!

Special thanks must be extended to my coworkers and colleagues who volunteered their time to read and provide comments on earlier versions of this work. Thank you Susan Amberg, AuD, Cathi Hayes, AuD, Elina Mindlina, AuD, Linsey Sunderhaus, AuD, Andrea Hedley-Williams, AuD, and Ally Sisler-Dinwiddie, AuD. You are all amazingly talented clinicians and I learn so much from each of you every day.

Finally, and most importantly, I want to thank my family, to whom I am completely committed (despite the fact that my laptop and I may be inseparable). My sons Levi, Jacob, and Aidan are a patient lot. If I had a dollar for every time they asked, "Are you still working on your book?" we'd have a pretty impressive pile of cash. Nevertheless, my boys have been supportive and are actually excited that Mom wrote a book—even if it is a "boring textbook." My husband, Branden, is the best husband this crazy, unorganized woman could ever have imagined. I am absolutely certain that he was handpicked for me by a higher power and I hope that he accepts both my thanks for his love and support and my apologies for working around the clock for much longer than initially anticipated.

Contributors

Deb Arthur, MA
Vice-President, Regulatory and Quality
Cochlear Americas
Chapter 1

Emily Lund, MS, CCC-SLP
PhD Candidate and Research Assistant
Department of Hearing and Speech Sciences
Vanderbilt University School of Medicine
Chapters 4 and 8

Patricia B. Macy, MA
Vice President Risk Management
MED-EL Corporation
Chapter 1

Cedric Navarro
Vice-President, Regulatory and Clinical Affairs
Advanced Bionics
Chapter 1

I believe in cochlear implants like I believe that the sun will rise and set each day. One cannot witness the life-altering outcomes for the recipients and their families and not believe in the power of this technology! My passion for this technology is rivaled only by my enthusiasm for the fields of audiology, speech-language pathology, otology, and deaf education. I know of no other line of work employing a more dedicated and impassioned group of professionals working toward the common goal of providing the best possible care for these precious patients and students. It is nothing short of a blessing to be granted the opportunity to work with cochlear implant recipients and their families. Every single patient has impacted me in his or her own special way. They have educated, humbled, and inspired me daily, and it is these special individuals who have motivated me to begin, and more importantly to finish this book. If this work furthers the education of a single student, clinician, teacher, patient, or parent, then I will consider my efforts meaningful. Thus, this work is dedicated to all cochlear implant recipients—young and old—and the professionals who devote their time and talent to ensure the highest possible outcomes.

1

FDA Candidacy for Cochlear Implantation

René H. Gifford, Cedric Navarro, Patricia B. Macy, and Deb Arthur

INTRODUCTION

The process of obtaining United States Food and Drug Administration (FDA) approval for biomedical devices is generally a foreign process to the working clinician; however, this process affects every clinician working with cochlear implant recipients. There are a number of misconceptions about FDA criteria for cochlear implantation, FDA labeling indications for adults and children, and how these affect the clinician's role in determining implant candidacy. Chapter 1 describes aspects concerning FDA approval for biomedical devices including the nature of the approval process, manufacturer-initiated clinical trials required for approval, as well as the role of the FDA in the regulation of biomedical devices. The chapter concludes with descriptions of the current FDA-labeled criteria for both adult and pediatric populations.

COCHLEAR IMPLANTS: FDA-REGULATED BIOMEDICAL DEVICES

The FDA is responsible for protecting public health by assuring that certain products are safe and effective, as well as monitoring such products for continued safety. The mission of the FDA is specifically listed as having the "responsibility of protecting the public health by assuring the safety, efficacy and security of human and veterinary drugs, biologic products, medical devices, our nation's food supply, cosmetics, and products that emit radiation" (FDA, 2012). To carry out this mission, the FDA is organized into a variety of centers and offices, each of which is focused on specific technologies.

The center that is responsible for overseeing medical devices, such as cochlear implants and hearing aids, is the Center of Devices and Radiological Health (CDRH). The CDRH device center regulates all companies that manufacture or import devices in the United States. The CDRH comprises several offices which each play a role in the regulation of medical devices. Those offices and their areas of responsibility and roles within the CDRH are shown in Table 1–1.

The U.S. Congress enacted the Medical Device Amendments of 1976 in order to "provide for the safety and effectiveness of medical devices intended for human use." The Medical Device Amendments were added to the Federal Food, Drug, and Cosmetic Act (FD&C Act), which was originally passed in 1938. The Medical Device Amendments established three regulatory classes for medical devices based on the degree of control necessary to ensure safety and effectiveness: classes I, II, and III.

Class I devices require that the device manufacturer provide the FDA with premarket notification, registration and listing, prohibitions against adulteration and misbranding, and rules for good manufacturing practices. Examples of Class I devices are elastic bandages, stethoscopes, nonpowered wheelchairs, hospital beds, and hearing aids.

Class II devices have the same requirements as Class I devices but additionally require that the manufacturer provide the FDA with performance standards. Examples of Class II devices are powered wheelchairs, surgical drapes, x-ray equipment, and osseointegrated hearing implant systems (e.g., Baha).

Class III devices have the same requirements as Class I and II devices but additionally require premarket approval (PMA). PMA is the required process of FDA scientific review to ensure safety and effectiveness of the device. Class III devices are those that support or sustain human life, prevent impairment of human health, and that may present a potentially unreasonable risk of illness or injury to the recipient (FDA, 2012). Examples of Class III devices are implantable pacemakers, implanted neuromuscular stimulators, and cochlear implants; thus, cochlear implants are placed in the most highly regulated category of medical devices.

In order to obtain PMA, cochlear implant manufacturers must submit an application to the CDRH for review and consideration (see Table 1–1). The FDA has specific branches within the Office of Device Evaluation (ODE) (Table 1–1), each having the knowledge and professional expertise to review the specific applications. Cochlear implants, middle ear implants, osseointegrated hearing implant systems, and hearing aids are the responsibility of the ODE Ear, Nose, and Throat branch. The reviewers in this branch are audiologists, hearing scientists, engineers, and

Table 1–1. Responsibilities of the Offices of the Center of Devices and Radiological Health

Office Name	Area of Responsibility
Office of Device Evaluation (ODE)	Approval of Class III devices
	Approval of investigational device exemptions required to collect clinical data in support of a device application
Office of Compliance (OC)	Review and approval of manufacturing and quality-control changes for Class III devices
	Enforces compliance to FDA regulations
Office of Science and Engineering Laboratories (OSEL)	Scientific review of Class II device applications when requested by either ODE or OC
	Provides scientific input to guidance documents and policy decisions
Office of Surveillance and Biometrics (OSB)	Monitors safety and efficacy of medical devices after they have been put on the market

ENT physicians/surgeons. ODE review panels can be composed of both FDA employees as well external consultants.

FDA REVIEW PROCESS FOR COCHLEAR IMPLANTS

New Devices

For new cochlear implant internal devices, processors, or significant design changes to internal and/or external devices, the implant manufacturers must submit a PMA application to the FDA which is reviewed by the ODE Ear, Nose and Throat branch for consideration. If the ODE reviewers decide that a more detailed scientific review is required in order to determine the safety and efficacy of the product in question, a request will be made for further review by staff from the Office of Science and Engineering Laboratories (OSEL). The OSEL has a staff of scientific reviewers who support all types of medical devices and associated technologies. For cochlear implants, there are OSEL reviewers with specialties in material sciences, mechanical engineering, neurophysiology, and hermeticity.

Existing Devices

If the cochlear implant manufacturers institute changes to manufacturing and/or quality control for existing devices that affect safety or efficacy, the Office of Compliance (OC) must be notified prior to the initiation of those changes. The OC reviews the proposal and can also request a detailed scientific review by OSEL staff. This review may include a site visit by the FDA in order to evaluate the new process of manufacturing and/or quality control in the manufacturing plant. The OC is also responsible for determining whether a manufacturer is in compliance with applicable legal requirements for manufacturing the devices, monitors device recalls, and performs regular facility inspections.

The final office of the CDRH shown in Table 1–1 is the Office of Surveillance and Biometrics (OSB) which is responsible for the evaluation and trending of medical device reports (MDRs). MDRs can be filed by manufacturers, patients, and/or health care providers for medical device failures or adverse events that result in harm; thus, the OSB reviews MDRs for existing devices.

FDA FUNDING

The FDA application, review, and monitoring of medical devices is intensive both in terms of the required time and personnel. Although these processes were put in place to ensure the safety and efficacy of devices for the American consumer, limited governmental funding is provided in order to carry out its mission and all associated responsibilities. In 2010, the U.S. Congress allocated approximately $3.18 billion for the FDA's annual budget. According to U.S. census bureau data, the national population in 2010 was 308,745,538; thus, the 2010 FDA budget amounted to just over $10 allocated for each individual living in the U.S. to carry out all responsibilities related to its mission. An obvious question centers on the feasibility of the FDA completing all of its assigned tasks and responsibilities in order to protect and promote public safety on such as limited budget. The answer to this question lies in the Medical Device User Fee and Modernization Act.

In 2002, the Medical Device User Fee and Modernization Act (MDUFMA), PL 107-250, was passed to amend the FD&C Act. The most significant provision of the MDUFMA—and that which is most relevant for cochlear implant manufacturers—was that which allowed the FDA to collect user fees for certain premarket reviews. Those PMAs subject to a user fee in accordance with MDUFMA include original PMAs, premarket reports, product development protocols, panel-track supplements, 180-day supplements, and real-time supplements. The user fees are updated annually and are available to the public on the FDA's website. Table 1–2 lists the 2012 medical device user fees most applicable for cochlear implant manufacturers.

Table 1–2. The 2012 Medical Device User Fees Most Applicable for Cochlear Implant Manufacturers

Application Type	Standard Fee (US$)	Small Business Fee (US$)
Premarket approval (PMA)	220,050	55,013
Panel-track PMA supplement	165,038	41,259
180-day PMA supplement	33,008	8,252
Real-time PMA supplement	15,404	3,851
30-day notice	3,521	1,760
Annual fee for periodic reporting on a class III device	7,702	1,925

DEVICE MODIFICATIONS REQUIRING FDA PMA APPROVAL

It is not the case that user fees are required only when first bringing a cochlear implant to market. Rather, PMA supplements are required in many cases when existing products are modified. One could argue that such tight regulation has the potential to inhibit product growth and development in the field of cochlear implants; however, the FDA explicitly states that the *least burdensome approach* should be taken in all areas of medical device regulation. It is this least burdensome approach to regulation that has prompted the development of multiple avenues for supplemental PMA.

A panel-track PMA is a supplement to an already approved PMA for which the manufacturer is requesting a "significant change in design or performance of the device, or a new indication for use of the device, and for which clinical data will be necessary to provide a reasonable assurance of safety and effectiveness" (FDA, 2008). For example, any time that the implant manufacturers revise indications or criteria for implantation, they are required to complete a clinical trial which itself requires FDA approval via investigational device exemption (IDE). Once the IDE is approved, the study is carried out at a number of medical centers across the country. Following completion

of the study, the manufacturer would then submit an application to the FDA for approval of the revised indications via a panel-track PMA supplement. This process is time and personnel intensive and quite costly to the manufacturer. It is for these reasons that the manufacturers do not regularly attempt to revise their indications for implantation despite the widespread knowledge that individuals with less severe hearing losses and better speech recognition scores, as well as children under 12 months of age, benefit from cochlear implants, and that broadening the criteria would allow more individuals with significant hearing loss to take advantage of the technology.

Manufacturers are required to submit a 180-day PMA supplement if they intend to make significant changes that affect the safety and effectiveness of the device. Manufacturer-requested changes to components, materials, design, specification, software, color additives, or labeling are considered appropriate for 180-day supplements. In some cases, the FDA may determine that the requested changes are sufficiently complex requiring a full PMA review by an outside advisory panel. In other cases, the FDA may determine that the proposed changes are minor and thus a real-time supplement may apply. A real-time supplement is one during which the supplement application is reviewed during a meeting or conference call and requires the review of only one scientific discipline.

The cochlear implant manufacturers are required to submit a 30-day notice when they plan to make changes to the manufacturing procedure or changes in the manufacturing method that could affect the safety and effectiveness of their device. A 30-day notice is sufficient as long as the changes do not alter performance or design specifications or the designated physical or chemical specifications of a device. Changes to the manufacturing procedure or method of manufacturing that do not affect the safety or effectiveness of the device must be submitted in the periodic report submitted to the FDA that is usually referred to as an annual report.

If a 30-day notice contains device-design or labeling changes in addition to manufacturing changes, the submission will automatically be converted to a 180-day PMA. If the change qualifies for a 30-day notice and complete information has been submitted, the device may be distributed 30 days after the date on which the FDA received the notice. If the information submitted is not adequate, within 30 days of receipt the FDA will provide notice that a 135-day PMA supplement is needed and will describe the additional information or action required for acceptance of the change. If no action occurs within 30 days of the FDA's receipt of the 30-day notice and payment of the user fee, the device may be distributed without further action from the FDA.

LABELED INDICATIONS FOR COCHLEAR IMPLANTATION AND OFF-LABEL USAGE

Current cochlear implant labeled indications (i.e., candidacy criteria) are listed in the physician's package insert that can be found in the packaging of each internal device. Contrary to popular belief, the FDA is *not* responsible for designating the criteria (indications) for cochlear implantation. Rather, the manufacturers submit an application for PMA outlining the indications for their device; thus, it is the role of the FDA to either approve or reject the submitted application for PMA and the manufacturer-defined indications. If ultimately approved, the manufacturer-defined indications for implantation are then listed as the FDA criteria for use of that device. These criteria are often referred to as the FDA labeled indications or FDA candidacy criteria; however, the indications are *approved* by the FDA but not set by the FDA.

What is important for the clinician to recognize in this process is that the FDA governs industry, not the individual clinician nor implant center. The industry—or in this case, the cochlear implant manufacturer—is strictly prohibited from promoting any off-label usage of its device. As is discussed in Chapter 5, despite considerable evidence in support of expanded cochlear implant candidacy criteria, the implant manufacturers are simply not permitted to recommend implantation for individuals not meeting all labeled indications. Clinicians, however, are granted the professional judgment to make clinical determinations for their patients about the suitability of cochlear implant candidacy. In fact, the FDA has provided an information sheet entitled "Off-Label and Investigational Use Of Marketed Drugs, Biologics, and Medical Devices" (FDA, 2011) which details the conditional approval of off-label usage of medical devices, drugs, and biologics as recommended by licensed clinicians. This information sheet explicitly endorses the off-label usage of a marketed medical device when the intent is for clinical practice and not for research purposes. The FDA (FDA, 2011) counsels that if clinicians recommend off-label usage of a medical device, they have the responsibility to ensure that the following three conditions are met:

1. Be well informed about the product.
2. Base its use on firm scientific rationale and on sound medical evidence.
3. Maintain records of the product's use and effects.

Off-label usage is nothing new in pharmaceuticals, biologics, and medical devices. For pharmaceuticals, estimates are that 20–60% are routinely prescribed for off-label usage across all medical specialties (e.g., Valeo, 2011; Jansen, 2011; Van Allen, Miyake, Gunn, Behler, & Kohlwes, 2011). In fact, the U.S. Supreme court ruled that off-label use of medical devices is an "accepted and necessary corollary of the FDA's mission" and that clinicians can "prescribe or administer any legally marketed device to a patient without limitation or interference" (Buckman Company v. Plaintiffs' Legal Committee, 2001).

Clinicians may discuss off-label use with individual patients and with colleagues in clinic and at scientific conferences; however, they are not allowed to advertise or market off-label usage to the general public. Such advertising would constitute a violation of the FD&C Act, which states that "a licensed practitioner may not promote a medical device for use(s) for which they have not received FDA clearance." For example, if a cochlear implant center took out an ad stating that individuals with mild to moderate hearing loss might benefit from cochlear implants and should thus consider coming into the center for evaluation, this would be direct violation of FDA policy.

Off-label usage of medical devices has become such common practice that even the Tennessee appellate court has ruled that this could be considered "standard of care" (Richardson v. Miller,

2000). Despite the ubiquity of off-label device usage across all fields, what remains critical is that we as clinicians respect the FDA's position on the stance of off-label cochlear implantation (FDA, 2011) and consider each patient's needs individually with our colleagues and members of the interdisciplinary cochlear implant team.

CURRENT COCHLEAR IMPLANT CRITERIA FOR ADULTS AND CHILDREN

Cochlear implant criteria, also referred to as labeled indications for cochlear implantation, have been set independently and differently by each of the cochlear implant manufacturers. The current adult and pediatric implant criteria at the time of writing are shown in Tables 1–3 and 1–4, respectively.

Note that there is considerable variability across the manufacturers for both adult and pediatric candidacy. In Table 1–3, for adult indications,

Table 1–3. Labeled Indications for Adult Cochlear Implantation as Shown for Advanced Bionics, Cochlear Americas, MED-EL, and CMS.

Adult Indications	Audiometric Thresholds	Speech-Recognition Performance
Advanced Bionics HR90K	Severe-to-profound bilateral sensorineural hearing loss (> 70 dB HL)	50% or less on a test of open-set sentence recognition (HINT sentences)
Cochlear Americas CI24RE CI512 CI422	Moderate-to-profound hearing loss in the low frequencies and profound ($\geq$ 90 dB HL) hearing loss in the mid to high speech frequencies	50% correct or less in the ear to be implanted (60% or less in the best-aided listening condition) on recorded tests of open-set sentence recognition
MED-EL PULSAR$_{CI}$100 SONATA$_{TI}$100 CONCERT	Bilateral severe-to-profound sensorineural hearing loss determined by a pure-tone average of 70 dB HL or greater at 500, 1000, and 2000 Hz	40% correct or less in best-aided listening condition on recorded tests of open-set sentence recognition (HINT sentences)
Centers for Medicare/Medicaid Services (CMS) National Coverage Determination	Bilateral moderate-to-profound sensorineural hearing loss	40% correct or less in best-aided listening condition on recorded tests of open-set sentence recognition

HINT Hearing in Noise Test

Table 1–4. Labeled Indications for Cochlear Implantation for Pediatric Implant Recipients as Shown for Advanced Bionics, Cochlear, and MED-EL

Pediatric Indications	Audiometric Thresholds	Auditory Skills and Speech Recognition		Amplification Requirements
		Younger Children	Older Children	
Advanced Bionics HR90K	Severe-to-profound bilateral sensorineural hearing loss (>70 dB HL)	**<4 years of age:** failure to reach developmentally appropriate auditory milestones (such as spontaneous response to name in quiet or to environmental sounds) measured using the Infant–Toddler Meaningful Auditory Integration Scale or Meaningful Auditory Integration Scale, or <20% correct on a simple open-set word-recognition test (Multisyllabic Lexical Neighborhood test [MLNT]) administered using monitored live voice (70 dB SPL)	**>4 years of age:** <12% on a difficult open-set word recognition (Phonetically Balanced Kindergarten test) or < 30% on an open-set sentences (Hearing In Noise Test for Children) administered using recorded materials in the sound field (70 dB SPL)	Use of appropriately fitted hearing aids for at least 6 months in children 2–17 years, or at least 3 months in children 12–23 months of age. The minimum duration of hearing aid use is waived in the presence of ossification concerns.
Cochlear Americas CI24RE CI512 CI422	**12–23 months:** bilateral profound sensorineural hearing loss; **24 months to 18 years:** bilateral severe-to-profound sensorineural hearing loss	Lack of progress in the development of simple auditory skills as quantified on a measure such as the Meaningful Auditory Integration Scale or the Early Speech Perception test	Less than or equal to 30% correct on MLNT or Lexical Neighborhood test (LNT), depending on the child's cognitive and linguistic skills	Use of appropriate amplification and participation in intensive aural habilitation over a 3- to 6-month period.
MED-EL PULSAR$_{CI}$[100] SONATA$_{TI}$[100] CONCERT	Profound bilateral sensorineural hearing loss with thresholds of 90 dB HL or greater at 1000 Hz	Lack of progress in the development of simple auditory skills in conjunction with appropriate amplification	<20% correct on the MLNT or LNT, depending on cognitive ability and linguistic skills	Use of appropriate amplification and participation in intensive aural habilitation over a 3- to 6-month period. Radiologic evidence of cochlear ossification may justify a shorter trial with amplification.

Cochlear makes reference to differing speech-recognition criteria for the ear to be implanted versus the "best-aided condition." On the other hand, AB, MED-EL, and CMS reference speech-recognition performance in the best-aided condition. (Chapter 2 discusses more recent recommendations regarding individual ear testing and focusing on the ear to be implanted.)

In Table 1–4, for pediatric criteria, none of the manufacturers reference criteria based on the ear to be implanted. In fact, the labeled indications for pediatric candidacy are much more stringent than those listed for adult candidacy. (Chapter 3 discusses pediatric criteria in depth, and Chapter 5 covers those cases for which expanded criteria are warranted.)

Unlike speech recognition criteria, the contraindications for cochlear implantation are consistent across both manufacturer and recipient age. The contraindications for cochlear implantation are as follows:

- Hearing loss originating in the auditory nerve or central auditory pathway
- Active external or middle ear infections
- Cochlear ossification preventing electrode insertion
- Cochlear nerve deficiency
- Tympanic membrane perforations associated with recurrent middle ear infections
- Allergy and/or intolerance of device materials (i.e., medical grade silicone, platinum, and titanium)

In addition to the contraindications listed above, CMS lists an additional contraindication as lacking the cognitive ability to use auditory clues and/or unwillingness to undergo an extended program of rehabilitation.

CONCLUSION

Indications for cochlear implantation are different for all three cochlear implant manufacturers and different yet for individuals covered by Medicare. Considering pediatric candidates, indications vary both with the child's age and developmental state; thus, it is no wonder that determining implant candidacy is not a straightforward process for either adult or pediatric candidates.

It is expected that indications will broaden over time; however, as discussed in this chapter, the process by which industry modifies labeling is time intensive and expensive. The FDA has specified the provisions allowing for off-label usage of medical devices as determined medically necessary by licensed medical professionals. Of course, insurance restrictions exist for patients with government insurance and even some private, commercial insurance plans. Thus, if we are to offer this technology to the individuals who can derive significant communicative benefit, the implant industry will ultimately need to conduct FDA-approved clinical trials via IDE and a subsequent PMA supplement to change labeled indications. As stated in the Introduction, although the process of FDA approval for biomedical devices tends to be a foreign process for the working clinician, it undoubtedly affects our role in determining implant candidacy.

REFERENCES

Buckman Company v. Plaintiffs' Legal Committee, 531 U.S. 341, 350 (2001).

FDA. (2008). *Modifications to devices subject to premarket approval (PMA). The PMA supplement decision.* Retrieved June 1, 2012, from http://www.fda.gov/medicaldevices/deviceregulationandguidance/guidancedocuments/ucm089274.htm

FDA. (2011). *"Off-Label" and investigational use of marketed drugs, biologics, and medical devices.* Retrieved June 1, 2012, from http://www.fda.gov/Regulatory Information/Guidances/ucm126486.htm

FDA. (2012). *Medical devices: Premarket approval.* Retrieved June 1, 2012, from http://www.fda.gov/medicaldevices/deviceregulationandguidance/howtomarketyourdevice/premarketsubmissions/premarketapprovalpma/default.htm

Jansen, R. M. (2011). Dissemination of information on the off-label (unapproved) use of medication: A comparative analysis. *Medical Law, 30*(1), 115–132.

Richardson v. Miller, 44 S.W.3d 1, 13, n.11 (Tenn. Ct. App. 2000).

Valeo, T. (2011). A Catch-22: Neurologists can prescribe off-label, but risk health insurers' denials for reimbursement. *Neurology Today, 11*(7), 28–30.

Van Allen, E. M., Miyake, T., Gunn, N., Behler, C. M., & Kohlwes, J. (2011). Off-label use of rituximab in a multipayer insurance system. *Journal of Oncology Practice, 7*(2), 76–79.

2

Adult Cochlear Implant Candidate Selection

René H. Gifford

INTRODUCTION

Cochlear implant criteria have evolved rapidly since the Food and Drug Administration (FDA) first approved multichannel cochlear implants for adults in 1985. Candidacy criteria vary with patient age, etiology of hearing loss, type of insurance coverage, and even across the different implant manufacturers. Further obscuring the determination of candidacy is the presence of overlapping indications with cochlear implants, hearing aids, osseous integrated auditory prostheses, middle ear implants, and shorter electrode, *atraumatic* cochlear implants for hearing preservation (i.e., Nucleus Hybrid and MED-EL electric and acoustic stimulation, EAS). With all these variables at play, the selection of appropriate cochlear implant candidates can be a complicated process—even for the most knowledgeable members of a cochlear implant team. On the other hand, clinicians who do not regularly work with cochlear implants may not be fully aware of how many patients can potentially benefit from this technology.

There are a number of aspects requiring consideration in the process of adult cochlear implant candidate selection. Although many are related to the audiologic evaluation including audiometric and speech recognition testing, there are also medical, radiologic, and psychological issues requiring careful consideration.

This chapter discusses the process of adult cochlear implant candidate selection including aspects to be considered from the perspective of the audiologist, speech/language pathologist, social worker and/or psychologist, as well as the medical/surgical team.

AUDIOLOGIC EVALUATION

Assessment of Hearing Status

Virtually all cochlear implant evaluations begin in the audiology clinic. By the time an adult patient is referred for a cochlear implant evaluation, they have likely already been followed for a number of years by an audiologist for hearing aid fittings. These patients have also likely been seen by an otolaryngologist for hearing aid medical clearance; thus, by the time an adult patient arrives for a cochlear implant evaluation, he or she is typically aware that hearing aids are not providing adequate benefit for successful communication and is ready to take the next step. From a professional perspective, this is generally a much different experience from that commonly faced by the rehabilitative audiologist recommending hearing aids—where denial and hesitation are often the norm.

Despite the fact that most patients present to the cochlear implant evaluation with prior audiograms, it is recommended that comprehensive audiometric testing be completed. This includes obtaining air-conduction thresholds for octave frequencies 125 through 8000 Hz as well as bone conduction, immittance, and standard speech audiometry (i.e., ear-specific speech-reception thresholds and word recognition). Obtaining thresholds at 125 Hz is particularly important given that the professions of otology and audiology are increasingly aware of minimally traumatic surgical techniques and low-frequency hearing preservation following cochlear implantation (e.g., Carlson et al., 2011; Gantz et al., 2009; Gstoettner et al., 2008; Skarzynski, Lorens, Piotrowska, & Anderson, 2006); thus, having this baseline information is critical if we are to investigate the presence of residual acoustic hearing in the implanted ear following surgery.

While OAEs are a valuable part of diagnostic audiology, they are generally not included in most adult implant evaluation protocols. The reason is that adult patients presenting for a cochlear implant evaluation will generally have been wearing hearing aids for a number of years. In fact, limited benefit from "appropriately fitted hearing aids" is listed as a requirement for determination of candidacy by all three cochlear implant manufacturers (Cochlear Americas package insert, Advanced Bionics package insert, MED-EL package insert). Thus, even if an adult had present OAEs at lower frequencies in the past, the use of amplification has been shown to be associated with secondary loss of OAEs per long-term use (Deltenre et al., 1999).

Cochlear Implant Criteria: Audiometric Thresholds

As discussed in Chapter 1, adult cochlear implant criteria differ across implant manufacturers. Audiometric criteria also differ across the manufacturers as well as across insurance carriers. Advanced Bionics and MED-EL specify bilateral severe-to-profound sensorineural hearing loss for adult implant candidacy (HR90K Physicians package insert, Sonata package insert). On the other hand, both Cochlear Americas and Medicare (Centers for Medicare & Medicaid Services [CMS], 2005) specify bilateral moderate-to-profound sensorineural hearing loss—recognizing that individuals with sloping hearing losses do not always obtain benefit from amplification allowing for successful communication. A common question posed by clinicians focuses on determination of candidacy for an individual who may meet the more relaxed audiometric criteria for Cochlear Americas and Medicare, but who may actually wish to pursue implantation with either Advanced Bionics or MED-EL. Though every implant program and team should develop their own protocol to address such matters, it is generally the case that if a patient meets implant candidacy criteria for any of the manufacturers, the patient is free to choose an implant system that meets their needs.[1] As stated in Chapter 1, FDA-labeled indications are provided as *guidelines* for device use and should not supersede professional clinical judgment.

SPEECH-RECOGNITION TESTING

Sensation Versus Perception

We were taught in Psychology 101 that there is a distinct difference between sensation and perception. Sensation is a lower-order sensory process by which an individual detects the presence of a stimulus in his or her environment. The audiogram is a perfect example of *sensation* in that audiometric thresholds represent a patient's *sen-*

---

[1]This does not apply to Medicare patients, because it is strongly recommended that CMS guidelines be strictly followed for all Medicare-insured patients.

sation or detection of the pure-tone stimuli. Perception, on the other hand, involves higher-order processing in that the sensed stimulus is sent to the brain for interpretation and derived meaning. Speech recognition testing is a perfect example of *perception* in that the patient's score represents the perception, recognition, and understanding of the presented speech stimulus.

In audiology, we have historically placed a lot of emphasis on the audiogram or the patient's *sensation* of tonal stimuli. While the audiogram serves as an excellent diagnostic tool, it provides limited information because it does not provide any data about the patient's functional *perception* of speech, and hence, his or her ability to communicate in everyday life. We have all heard patients report that they can hear (sensation) but that they just cannot understand (perception). Furthermore, it is well recognized that similar audiograms can yield very different functional outcomes with respect to speech perception abilities; thus, it is critical for us clinicians to consider a patient's complete audiologic profile so that we avoid the trap of failing to look *beyond* the audiogram.

Speech-Perception Metrics

Much of the preoperative assessment in this section can also be found in the Minimum Speech Test Battery (MSTB). The MSTB was originally developed in 1996 when representatives from the American Academy of Otolaryngology—Head and Neck Surgery, the American Academy of Audiology, and an experienced group of clinicians/scientists from the cochlear implant manufacturers met to determine the MSTB recommended for audiologic cochlear implant candidacy and for longitudinal assessment of postoperative performance. The MSTB manual, which was revised in 2011 and is frequently referenced throughout this book, can be downloaded for free at http://www.auditorypotential.com/MSTB.html.

Recorded Materials

A central component of all adult cochlear implant evaluations is the behavioral assessment of speech recognition. Many individuals with hearing loss report that in order to "hear," they must be able to "see" the talker, that is, they rely heavily—if not entirely—on visual cues such as lip reading and more global nonverbal communication; thus, in order to gain an understanding of an individual's auditory-based, speech recognition abilities, stimuli must be presented without visual cues.

The most important aspect surrounding the administration of speech stimuli involves the use of recorded speech materials. The use of recorded materials for speech recognition assessment has been recommended since 1949 when the Father of Audiology, Raymond Carhart (1949), suggested that the use of a phonograph recording would increase the test stability across conditions. Unfortunately, however, over two-thirds of audiologists report that they routinely use monitored live voice (MLV) for administration of speech recognition materials (Martin, Champlin, & Chambers, 1998; Medwetsky, Sanderson, & Young, 1999). It is unclear, however, whether this estimate included audiologists involved in determining cochlear implant candidacy.

Roeser and Clark (2008) examined word recognition performance obtained with recorded materials as compared with MLV for 32 ears. As shown in Figure 2–1, Roeser and Clark reported that word recognition scores for MLV and recorded stimuli were significantly different for 23 of the 32 ears (or 72% of the population). In fact, the difference between the scores obtained via MLV and recorded stimuli was as high as 80 percentage points; thus, these data confirm the critical need for the elimination of MLV presentation particularly for the assessment of cochlear implant candidacy. Currently, Cochlear Americas, MED-EL, and CMS specify the use of recorded stimuli for the implant evaluation. The prevalence of recorded materials available on both compact disc as well as digitized for transmission from the output of the computer sound card directly to the audiometer makes for simple and inexpensive use as well as presentation.

Presentation Level

A second critical aspect of speech recognition testing for cochlear implant evaluations involves the presentation level of the recorded speech stimuli. For many years the accepted presentation level for

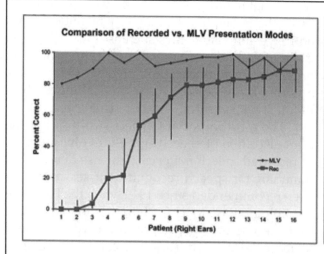
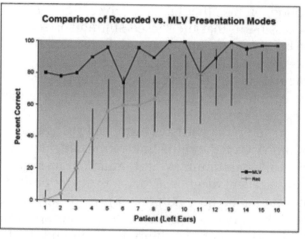

FIGURE 2–1. Comparison of word-recognition scores for the right ear (**A**) and left ear (**B**) using monitored live voice and recorded presentation for 16 patients. The ranges shown for the recorded presentations are the 95% confidence levels predicted from the binomial tables of Raffin and Thorton (1980). Reprinted with permission.

the stimulus was 70 dB SPL because this was thought to be necessary in order to provide audibility for individuals with severe-to-profound hearing loss. The problem with using a presentation level of 70 dB SPL is that it is not representative of average, conversational-level speech. In a study funded by the Environmental Protection Agency, Pearsons, Bennett, and Fidell (1977) reported that average conversational speech was 60 dB SPL, and that 70 dB SPL was (1) representative of raised level or loud speech and (2) not sustainable from a talker's perspective for an extended period of time. A number of studies have evaluated speech perception performance for both pre-implant (Alkaf & Firszt, 2007) and post-implant recipients (Firszt et al., 2004; Skinner, Holden, Holden, Demorest, & Fourakis, 1997) at multiple presentation levels including 50, 60, and 70 dB SPL. They found that postoperative performance for both 60 and 70 dB SPL were essentially identical but that *preoperative* performance was significantly poorer for 60 dB SPL as compared with 70 dB SPL; thus, using 70 dB SPL as the presentation level is not appropriate for determining implant candidacy because it (1) puts the individual at a disadvantage because

it is not representative of average conversational levels in the real world, (2) has the potential to artificially inflate one's speech recognition performance, and (3) may disqualify an individual from candidacy who could derive significant benefit from cochlear implantation.

Both Cochlear Americas (Balkany et al., 2007) and Advanced Bionics (FDA NCT01066780, 2010) have recently completed clinical trials which have incorporated a 60-dB-SPL level (A weighting) for presentation of speech stimuli; thus, best practices recommendations as included in the 2011 MSTB manual have included the use of recorded speech materials presented at 60 dBA[2] for assessment of speech recognition performance for pre- as well as post-implant testing.

Speech Recognition Test Materials for Determining Candidacy in Adults

A variety of speech recognition materials are available to be used in the assessment of cochlear implant candidacy including monosyllabic words, sentences, and sentences in noise. With respect

---

[2]The use of A weighting for sound-level-meter measurements is recommended due to the fact that linear weighting, which is implied in an SPL reference unless otherwise specified, provides noisier recordings due to flat frequency response through the lower-frequency region. In contrast, the A-weighted frequency response rolls off for lower frequencies having reached 20 dB of attenuation, relative to pass-band, at 100 Hz.

to adult cochlear implant candidacy, the MSTB committee recommended that speech recognition performance be assessed with both monosyllabic words (consonant nucleus consonant [CNC] words) (Peterson & Lehiste, 1962) and the Hearing in Noise Test (HINT) sentences (Nilsson, Soli, & Sullivan, 1994) presented in quiet and in a fixed-level noise background. Although the MSTB committee did not specify a criterion performance level for determining implant candidacy, they recommended that "at each preoperative and postoperative evaluation, one 50-word CNC list and two 10-sentence HINT lists should be presented in quiet." The committee also recommended that the HINT sentences be presented in fixed-level noise at +10, +5, or even 0 dB signal-to-noise ratio (SNR) as necessary to avoid ceiling effects (Nilsson, McCaw, & Soli, 1996). Despite these recommendations, current adult cochlear implant candidacy in the United States, with respect to speech recognition performance, is based *solely* on sentence recognition in a quiet background. Generally, the HINT sentences are presented in quiet and used for qualification purposes. Cochlear Americas and CMS, however, do not specify a sentence metric but rather refer to open-set, sentence recognition materials for determining candidacy.

As with the other previously discussed aspects of implant candidacy, each manufacturer outlines a slightly different set of indications found in the FDA-approved Physician's Package Insert labeling for each device. At the time of chapter preparation, Advanced Bionics specified HINT sentence recognition up to 50% in the best-aided condition. Cochlear Americas specified sentence recognition up to 50% correct in the ear to be implanted and up to 60% in the best-aided condition. MED-EL listed HINT sentence recognition up to 40% correct in the best-aided condition. Lastly, CMS criteria were also outlined independently to include sentence recognition up to 40% correct in the best-aided condition.

Recently a committee of audiologist clinician/scientists convened to discuss the assessment of speech perception for cochlear implant recipients (Fabry, Firszt, Gifford, Holden, & Koch, 2009). Based on clinical survey data and literature review, the committee recommended a speech perception test battery for assessing both pre- and post-implant performance. The recommended

test battery was estimated to take approximately 30–45 min to administer, which is an important consideration given the busy clinical environment. The recommended battery included CNC words, AzBio sentences (Spahr et al., 2012), and AzBio sentences presented in multitalker babble using a +5 dB SNR or one list pair of the Bamford-Kowal-Bench-Sentence-in-Noise (BKB-SIN) test (version 1.03, Etymotic Research, Inc.; Killion, Niquette, Revit, & Skinner, 2001). The recommended use of the AzBio sentences over the seemingly ubiquitous HINT sentences stemmed from the finding that the HINT sentences suffer from ceiling effects for post- and even some pre-implant individuals (Gifford, Shallop, & Peterson, 2008). In fact, the cochlear implant manufacturers in the United States have now moved to include the AzBio sentences in a new battery of tests that will serve as the standard for evaluation of pre- and post-implant assessments of speech recognition. The implant companies have recommended a test battery including AzBio sentences, BKB-SIN, and CNC monosyllabic words. The use of words, sentences in quiet, and sentences in noise provides information on the individual's performance in a variety of listening conditions as well as verification of subject performance via cross-checking across the different speech recognition materials and the known interrelationship of individual performance on those measures.

Hearing Aid Verification

Prior to the consideration of which speech metric should be used to determine candidacy, we must first verify that the patient has appropriately fitted hearing aids. This is particularly important since limited benefit from appropriately fitted hearing aids is specifically listed as a requirement for implant candidacy by all three cochlear implant manufacturers.

Verification of hearing aid settings may mean different things to different clinicians; however, there are clearly defined practice guidelines for verifying hearing aid settings. In 2006, the American Academy of Audiology published the "Guidelines for the Audiologic Management of Adult Hearing Impairment" (Valente et al., 2006). These guidelines state that "prescribed gain from a validated prescriptive method should be verified using a probe-microphone approach that is referenced to ear canal SPL." What this means is that functional gain measures are *not* appropriate for verification of hearing aid settings as part of the candidacy selection process. Although aided sound field thresholds provide information about audibility of low-level stimuli, they do not provide data regarding audibility for the average conversational level speech, which is a benchmark of successful communication.

There are many options for the use of probe microphone measures in the verification of hearing aid settings, most of which are not only beyond the scope of this book but could also comprise an entire book on their own. One consideration for probe-microphone measurements that is closely related to the implant candidacy process, however, is the choice of level used for the verification of gain and/or output of the hearing aid. As mentioned previously, the MSTB recommends a presentation level of 60 dB SPL for speech stimuli used in the determination of implant candidacy; thus, it would follow that the stimulus used for hearing aid verification, whether it be speech or a speechlike signal, should also be 60 dB SPL. Verification at other levels may also be incorporated by individual implant program protocols; however, 60 dB SPL should be considered the level used in the verification of hearing aids and is considered the minimum required for best practices in hearing aid verification prior to determining implant candidacy. Despite the efficacy of cochlear implantation, it is of critical importance that candidacy be determined with appropriately fitted hearing aids to ensure that the least invasive treatment option be determined for all patients.

Testing Conditions

The testing conditions for determining cochlear implant candidacy are not widely agreed upon among clinicians. All three manufacturers use the term "best-aided condition" when referring to speech recognition performance for both adults and children. Medicare criteria also specify the "best-aided condition" as the performance to be considered for determining implant candidacy. Only one of the manufacturers, Cochlear Americas, specifically states different performance criteria for the ear to be implanted as compared with the best-aided listening condition, allowing for binaural summation and/or asymmetry between the ears. The problem is that "best-aided condition" is subject to interpretation. In the case of asymmetric hearing loss and/or speech recognition performance across the ears, the best-aided condition may be a gross overestimation of performance as compared with performance for the proposed ear to be implanted. Fabry et al. (2009) recommended individual ear testing for postoperative assessment of performance; thus, it would follow that we should be assessing individual ear performance preoperatively, as well. In fact, Cochlear Americas has received FDA approval to conduct a clinical trial examining new indications for adult cochlear implantation in which candidacy would be based on speech perception performance in the ear to be implanted. Given this, it is likely that more emphasis will be placed on assessing the ear to be implanted as well as a best-aided condition, and that ultimately, candidacy will be determined based on data for the ear to be implanted.

The MSTB released in 2011 does not specifically list recommendations for testing conditions to be used either pre- or postoperatively; thus, it is important for each cochlear implant program to determine a protocol based on the goals for preoperative testing. Given that it is reasonable to assume speech perception performance will be assessed for the cochlear implant-only condition postoperatively, it follows that individual ear performance must also be quantified preoperatively in order to have a baseline against which future gains in performance can be compared. It may be the case that not all speech metrics are presented to each ear individually as well as in the best-aided condition during the pre-implant workup; but it is of critical importance for determining individual implant efficacy that individual ear performance as well as the best-aided condition be assessed for at least one speech metric.[3]

---

[3]This does not apply to those ears for which there is no behavioral hearing—and hence no hearing aid can be worn—in the preoperative condition.

Testing Setup and Calibration

Testing for adult cochlear implant candidacy requires a sound-treated booth or room as well as a calibrated audiometer, loudspeaker, compact disc player, or computer[4] with sound card or MP3 player, and a comfortable chair for the patient. The sound-treated room should meet ANSI S3.1, American National Standard for Maximum Permissible Ambient Noise Levels for Audiometric Test Rooms (ANSI, 1999). In addition to minimizing ambient noise levels, it is important to minimize reflectant surfaces in the sound booth as reverberation is known to affect speech recognition.

The MSTB recommends that the loudspeaker be placed at a distance of approximately 1 m from the listener with the listener seated at or close to the center of the room. For that reason, the minimum room size required for preoperative implant candidacy evaluation is 1.83 × 1.83 m (6 × 6 feet). The reasoning behind the 1-m distance recommendation is related to the near/far-field boundary. When a signal is presented via a loudspeaker, there is an associated near field and far field. In the near field, large SPL changes are observed for small changes in distance from the loudspeaker. It is for this reason that sound-field testing is typically completed with listeners placed between the near/far-field boundary. For most audio sound booths, the distance between the listener and the loudspeaker tends to be approximately 1 m (Dirks, Morgan, & Wilson, 1976) and should not be close to the walls of the room or any other reflective surfaces.

The loudspeaker should be positioned at the level of a typical seated listener's head (approximately 39 inches [86 cm] from the floor) at 0° azimuth. Figure 2–2 shows an example of an adult cochlear implant recipient seated in an audiometric sound booth meeting all of the above-listed criteria.

Calibrating Speech Stimuli

Calibration of speech stimuli for presentation in the free field requires that both the input and out-

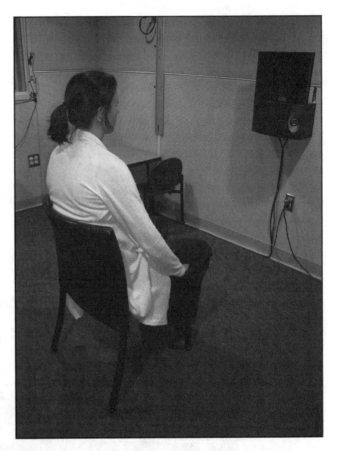

FIGURE 2–2. An adult cochlear implant recipient is seated at a distance of just over 1 meter from the speaker for speech recognition testing.

put of the audiometer be calibrated. Generally a calibration tone at 1000 Hz is provided along with the stimuli to calibrate the input level to the audiometer. To do this, set the audiometer to External A or B, corresponding to the input port used to connect to the CD player, MP3 player, or computer. The transducer is set to *speaker*, although it is not critical at this point as only the input is being calibrated; however, to avoid presentation of a high-level stimulus through the speaker—which, depending on the dial setting of the audiometer can be startling or even sufficiently loud to approach discomfort—it is recommended that the dial be set to a low level such as −10 dB HL. Next, the *interrupt* or *stimulus* button

---

[4]Should your clinic decide to upload digitized speech stimuli to a computer hard drive, it is still important to be cognizant of the site licenses required for individual speech tests. For example, if your clinic has three sound booths, then three copies of the material would still need to be purchased.

should be selected to present the input calibration tone through the audiometer. Once the calibration tone is on, the sensitivity dials for External A and/ or B are adjusted to ensure that the VU meter is set to 0 or just below. This is done to avoid distortion and clipping of the input signal.

Once the input signal is calibrated and the sensitivity dials of External A and/or B are set, these dials should *not* be adjusted further during the calibration and presentation process. Instead, calibration of the output signal through the loudspeaker to the desired presentation level is completed by manipulating the audiometer dial setting.

Calibration of the signal output requires the use of a sound level meter (SLM). The SLM microphone can be placed on a stand or suspended from the ceiling via cable so that the microphone is placed at the position of a typical listener's

head when the listener is seated in a chair. This MSTB manual recommends that this height be approximately 39 inches (86 cm) from the floor, which also corresponds to the recommended level of the loudspeaker. This method of calibration is referred to as the substitution method as the calibration does not involve probe tube microphone placement for the actual patient but instead involves the substitution of the SLM microphone at the approximate placement of the listener's head. Figures 2–3 and 2–4 display possible SLM microphone placements: on a stand or suspended from the ceiling via extension cable, respectively. The former method (see Figure 2–3) is recommended for clinics in which daily access to a SLM is not possible. The latter method (see Figure 2–4) is a convenient way to achieve daily calibration of the speech stimuli without having to move SLM equipment in and out of the booth. The use of

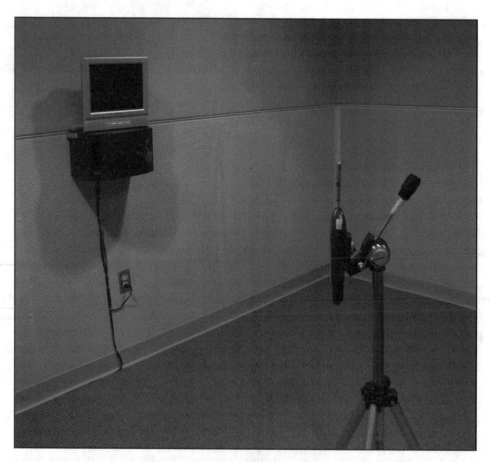

FIGURE 2–3. SLM microphone placement on a stand.

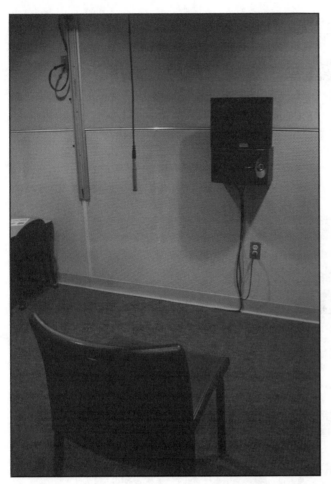

FIGURE 2–4. SLM microphone placement suspended from the ceiling via an extension cable.

an extension cable also allows for (1) placement of the SLM in the control room next to the audiometer for easy calibration without having to go back and forth between the control room and the booth until the desired output level is achieved, and (2) daily calibration and/or calibration prior to conducting sound field speech recognition testing for every patient. An extension cable can be used in conjunction with a mic stand so that the SLM can be located in the control room next to the clinician; however, this is not the norm.

A calibration noise accompanies speech stimuli on CD or via WAV or MP3 stimuli for sound field calibration. Setting the SLM to A weighting and fast response, adjust the audiometer dial in 1-dB increments until the display reads 60 dBA. It is at this dial setting, and accompanying EXT A/B sensitivity dial setting, that the speech stimuli will

also be presented at 60 dBA, which is the MSTB recommended presentation level.

Ideally speech stimuli presented in the sound field should be calibrated prior to each presentation or testing session. Unless the clinic owns a SLM dedicated for sound field calibration in a particular sound booth, this is not a realistic option. The next best option would be to complete daily calibration. Any schedule that does not involve calibration prior to each testing session runs the risk of inaccuracy. Using inaccurate presentation levels could lead to inappropriate recommendations regarding cochlear implant candidacy involving either under- or overqualifying patients. This is particularly true if a clinic is using digitized/computerized speech stimuli. The reason is that the output volume for the computer sound card directly influences the input to the audiometer and the level of the corresponding loudspeaker. For clinics using digitized/computerized stimuli, it is recommended that the master volume on the computer always be set to maximum. The computer volume setting should be *checked prior to each and every testing session*. It is critical to communicate to all clinicians in a given practice that the computer volume should not be adjusted.

Time Allotted for CIWU

How much time should be allotted for a cochlear implant evaluation or workup appointment? This depends on an individual clinic protocol. Some clinics may choose to follow MSTB recommendations for pre-implant workups but only include the minimum recommended testing schedule due to time, space, and/or personnel restrictions. Other clinics may choose to incorporate the MSTB recommendations but also obtain supplemental information during the workup with additional tests, metrics, and/or conditions. Using the MSTB's minimum recommended schedule as shown in Table 2–1, the approximate times for completion of each audiologic procedure were obtained from a time study of practice patterns for standard audiometry (Tucker, 2001) as well as for hearing aid verification (Busen & McCarthy, 2010). Time estimates for aided speech perception

Table 2–1. Minimum Recommended Schedule of the Minimum Speech Test Battery (Adult Candidacy Workup Checklist)

Comprehensive Audiologic Evaluation	
Audiometric thresholds (AC & BC)	AC: 125–8000 Hz
Speech audiometry	SRT and word recognition, recorded stimuli
Tympanometry	
Acoustic reflex thresholds	
Acoustic reflex decay (if possible)	
Hearing Aid (HA) Verification	
Electroacoustic verification and real ear measures	
Speech or speechlike stimuli at 60 dB SPL	
Aided Speech Recognition Testing	
Recorded stimuli, 60 dB SPL, best-aided condition[a]	
CNC	One 50-item list
AzBio sentences	One 20-sentence list
BKB-SIN test	One paired list
Administration of Questionnaires	
Expectations questionnaire(s)	
Preimplant administration of outcome measures and quality-of-life questionnaire(s)	

[a]At least one metric should also be administered in the right-HA and left-HA conditions

CNC consonant nucleus consonant; *SRTs* speech-reception thresholds; *BKB-SIN* Bamford-Kowal-Bench-Sentence-in-Noise

testing were obtained from the MSTB document itself. Table 2–2 provides time estimates for each of the procedures outlined in the MSTB. The estimates for audiometry and hearing aid verification reflect mean time estimates (in minutes) plus two standard deviations, as 95% of the expected values should fall within this range assuming a normal distribution. The time estimates for aided speech perception reflect the expected range of time (in minutes) needed for administration and scoring. Using the estimates provided in Table 2–2, the total time required for audiometric testing, hearing aid verification, and aided speech perception testing would range from 111 to 121 min. This time does not take into account the need to reprogram

hearing aids should the patient's own hearing aid settings not be providing target audibility.

Though this may seem like a lot of time for testing, it is reasonable to err on the conservative side. The reason is that the severity of hearing losses observed with pre-implant patients often necessitates written instructions on a large computer monitor facing the patient or by writing instructions on paper or dry erase board. For this reason, it is a good idea for each clinic to prepare simple written instructions for audiometry and speech perception testing that can be used at each cochlear implant evaluation.

In addition to the 111–121 min for testing completed during a cochlear implant evaluation,

Table 2–2. Time Estimates for Each of the Procedures Outlined in the Minimum Speech Test Battery (*MSTB*; Adult Candidacy Workup Checklist)

Procedure		Estimated Time (min)
Comprehensive audiometry (AC, BC, SRT, WR)		36.4
Tympanometry		6.8
Acoustic reflex thresholds		11.2
Acoustic reflex decay (if possible)		9.6
Hearing Aid (HA) Verification		
Electroacoustic verification and real ear measures		22.0
Aided Speech Recognition Testing		
Recorded stimuli, 60 dB SPL, best-aided condition		
CNC	One 50-item list	5–7 (MSTB)
AzBio sentences	One 20-sentence list	5–7 (MSTB)
BKB-SIN test	One paired list	5–7 (MSTB)
Recorded stimuli, 60 dB SPL, Individual ear testing		
CNC*	One 50-item list, per ear	10-14 (MSTB)

Administration of questionnaires (completed in waiting room or prior to visit)

*Choice of metric for individual ear testing may be determined by clinical protocol. An ideal environment would allow time for administration of all metrics for individual ears preoperatively to allow postoperative assessment of benefit as it is not always clear which ear will be implanted at the time of evaluation.

CNC consonant nucleus consonant; *SRT* speech-reception threshold; *BKB-SIN* Bamford-Kowal-Bench-Sentence-in-Noise

the clinician must allocate a significant portion of time for reviewing test results, questionnaires, counseling, and introduction of the available cochlear implant systems. Should the clinician have to type or write to the patient, this time is lengthened considerably; thus, it is reasonable to allocate approximately 3 hr for a cochlear implant evaluation.

SUBJECTIVE EVALUATION OF ADULT PRE-IMPLANT PERFORMANCE

Evidence-based practice (EBP) is gaining increasingly more attention in clinical patient care as insurance companies require proof of treatment efficacy for coverage purposes. EBP in audiology has largely been associated with hearing aid fit-tings; however, EBP plays an active role in the pre-implant evaluation and postoperative fitting and assessment of patients with cochlear implants, as well. Objective measures of postoperative speech perception and subjective assessments of perceived performance and/or benefit may not be in good agreement with one another (Wackym, Runge-Samuelson, Firszt, Alkaf, & Burg, 2007). One likely explanation is that the laboratory conditions assessed in the audiometric test booth may not truly reflect real-world listening conditions. Furthermore, subjective assessment instruments can also serve to validate the efficacy of a particular treatment option such as cochlear implantation. Although we recognize the efficacy of cochlear implantation with respect to restoration of hearing and speech recognition, we do not routinely assess the effect of cochlear implants on a recipient's social and/or emotional welfare or the more global effect on one's quality of life.

On another level, the use of subjective measures during the *preoperative* assessment can provide an element of information that is not necessarily contained within the objective scores of speech recognition.

There are a number of instruments used to assess subjective benefit, performance, and/or quality of life following cochlear implantation. Although the 24-item Abbreviated Profile of Hearing Aid Benefit (APHAB) (Cox & Alexander, 1995) was designed to gauge degree of benefit following hearing aid fittings, due to the ease of administration and the relative brevity of the questionnaire, it is often used in cochlear implant programs, as well. The APHAB self-assessment scale evaluates listening difficulties experienced in four areas: ease of communication, background noise, reverberation, and aversiveness of sound; thus, the difference in listening difficulties found pre- and post-implant provides an index of the benefit associated with cochlear implantation.

The Client-Oriented Scale of Improvement (COSI) (Dillon, James, & Ginis, 1997) is a clinical assessment instrument developed by National Acoustic Laboratories for evaluating individually determined outcomes following amplification. The COSI can be easily adapted for use with cochlear implant recipients as the patient can identify listening situations which he or she would like improvement with cochlear implants. Although the COSI is a great tool for use with patients, it is limited in its across-patient comparison due to the individual nature of the instrument.

The Nijmegen Cochlear Implant Questionnaire (NCIQ) (Hinderink, Krabbe, & Broek, 2000) is a 60-item, quality-of-life instrument designed for use with adult cochlear implant recipients. The NCIQ assesses six domains including basic sound perception (e.g., environmental sounds), advanced sound perception (e.g., modulation of one's own voice, speech intelligibility), speech perception, self-esteem, activity, and social interactions. The NCIQ was designed for administration both at pre- and post-implant assessments.

The 25-item Cochlear Implant Function Index (CIFI) (Coelho, Yeh, Kim, & Lalwani, 2009) is a self-assessment instrument that was designed and validated for use with adult cochlear implant recipients. The CIFI evaluates an individual's reliance on visual cues, use of the telephone, communication at work as well as hearing in noise, in groups, and in large-room settings. As with the other instruments, the CIFI is recommended for administration both pre- and post-implant.

The 18-item Glasgow Benefit Inventory (GBI) (Robinson, Gatehouse, & Browning, 1996) was developed to gauge patient benefit derived specifically from otorhinolaryngologic (ORL) surgical interventions. Specifically, the GBI defines patient benefit as the change in one's health status directly resulting from the procedure. The GBI questions were written to be independent of any particular diagnosis or intervention; thus, the degree of "benefit" across different ORL procedures could be compared. The inherent flexibility of the GBI can also be viewed as a weakness because it does not specifically address aspects that may be of interest to those undergoing cochlear implantation. The GBI would be administered post-implant as the 18 questions to address the change in state following the procedure such as, "Since your operation/intervention, do you have more or less self-confidence?" or "Since your operation/intervention, do you feel more or less confident about job opportunities?" Responses to GBI questions are based on a five-point Likert scale ranging from a large decline to large improvement in health status.

The Glasgow Hearing Aid Benefit Profile (GHABP) (Gatehouse, 1999) was designed to quantify hearing aid benefit as related to situations in which hearing-related handicap most likely exists. It includes assessment of difficulty and the benefits of a hearing aid for four fixed communicative situations including (1) listening to the television with family or friends when the volume is adjusted to suit other people, (2) having a conversation with one other person when there is no background noise, (3) carrying on a conversation in a busy street or shop, and (4) having a conversation with several people in a group. In addition to these four fixed situations, the GHABP allows for the patient to identify up to four additional situations in which he or she feels it is important to be able to hear as well as possible. Clinicians employing the GHABP in their Hearing Aid Program may find it also useful to use the GHABP in their Cochlear Implant Program with some modifications to the language to address implant(s) over hearing aid(s).

The Hearing Handicap Inventory for Adults (HHIA) (Newman, Weinstein, Jacobson, & Hug, 1990) and Hearing Handicap Inventory for the Elderly (HHI-E) (Ventry & Weinstein, 1982) both include 25 questions designed to gauge functional handicap resulting from hearing loss. Respondents answer yes (4 points), sometimes (2 points), or no (0 points) to questions such as *Does a hearing problem cause you to use the phone less often than you would like?* and *Does a hearing problem cause you to avoid groups of people?* Although the HHIA and HHIE were designed as a screening tool to quantify functional, day-to-day hearing difficulties, it may also be used as an outcome measure in a pre- versus post-treatment administration. Given that many clinics may already be using the HHIA/HHIE in the general audiology clinic or as part of the hearing aid clinic, post-implant administration could also be implemented.

More generic quality-of-life assessment instruments are also available and are widely used in cochlear implant research, though they may also be useful in the clinical environment. Health-related, quality-of-life questionnaires can assign a numerical value to duration of life as modified by the impairments (e.g., hearing loss), functional states, perceptions, and social opportunities that can be influenced by disease, injury, treatment, or policy (Patrick & Erickson, 1993). The Health Utilities Index (HUI) Mark III (Furlong, Feeny, Torrance, & Barr, 2001) is a multidimensional instrument that assesses individual abilities on attributes including vision, hearing, speech, ambulation, dexterity, emotion, cognition, and pain. There are multiple questionnaire formats available including self-assessment, clinician-administered, and even proxy-assessment versions. Although these tools were designed with a clinical research focus, one could reasonably incorporate such an instrument into clinical protocol for cochlear implant candidate selection and assessment of health-related changes following cochlear implantation.

In addition to questionnaires designed to track outcome measures and overall quality-of-

life changes resulting from cochlear implantation, there are also a number of expectation questionnaires that can be administered preoperatively. Pre-implant expectation questionnaires require patients to document, in writing, what they believe cochlear implants can provide for them in terms of benefit. Such questionnaires can be an integral part of the pre-implant evaluation because they facilitate patient-specific counseling—particularly in cases for which a patient may exhibit inappropriate expectations in his or her responses. Many clinics upload the questionnaire, along with signatures of both the patient and clinician and addressed comments, into the patient's electronic medical record. That way, the questionnaire and comments can later serve as a counseling tool should the patient express unrealistic post-implant expectations, particularly those that may differ from their pre-implant responses.

There are a number of available expectations questionnaires related specifically to cochlear implantation (Cochlear Corporation, 2003). The expectations questionnaires are organized into True/False questions that all begin with the statement, "When I am using the cochlear implant . . . " Examples of the questions include *Conversation over the telephone will be easy to understand* as well as *I can be assured of better job opportunities because of better hearing.*

ROLE OF THE SOCIAL WORKER AND/OR PSYCHOLOGIST IN THE DETERMINATION OF COCHLEAR IMPLANT CANDIDACY

The role of the social worker and/or psychologist in the determination of cochlear implant candidacy can be pivotal for adult recipients. Psychological evaluations are generally not routinely scheduled for adult cochlear implant evaluations as was the common practice when cochlear implants were first introduced clinically. Scheduling a visit with a psychologist and/or social worker in select adult cases, however, can provide valuable information for not only the cochlear implant team, but also for the patient and his or her family. For example, adult patients who were prelingually deafened as well as individuals who have had sudden onset profound hearing loss are obvious populations that could benefit from a preoperative psychological evaluation and/or appointment with a social worker specially trained to work with hearing-impaired individuals. The goal of the cochlear implant team is to evaluate each patient individually and recommend psychological and/or social worker attention for adult candidates on a case-by-case basis, as needed.

It is a well-known fact that hearing loss is associated with increased incidence of depression, social anxiety, loneliness, and overall psychological distress in the adult population (e.g., Abrams, Barnett, Hoth, Schultz, & Kaboli, 2006; Knutson, Johnson, & Murray, 2006; Nachtegaal et al., 2009; Gopinath et al., 2009). Although cochlear implantation has been shown to significantly reduce depression and other psychosocial symptoms in individuals with hearing loss (Knutson et al., 1998; Knutson et al., 1991; Olze et al., 2011; Poissant, Beaudoin, Huang, Brodsky, & Lee, 2008), it is possible that an individual seeking a cochlear implant may have unrealistic expectations regarding how much the implant will improve his or her depressive symptoms; thus, it is important for the clinician to refer individuals with reported depression and social anxiety related to one's hearing loss for preoperative psychological evaluation. Though there are a number of depression screening tools available, it is recommended that each cochlear implant team consult with the psychologist and/or psychiatrist on the cochlear implant team for recommendations.

MEDICAL AND SURGICAL EVALUATION: IMPLANT CANDIDATE SELECTION

The cochlear implant surgeon, a specialist in otology or neurotology, plays an obviously critical role in the determination of implant candidacy. Surgeons complete a thorough preoperative evaluation in addition to being responsible for the implant surgical procedure and postoperative otologic medical care. The otologist and his or her medical team ensure that all cochlear implant candidates are up to date on their immunizations prior to cochlear implantation. The recommended immunization schedule for adults can be found on the Centers for Disease Control website (http://www.cdc.gov/vaccines/vpd-vac/mening/cochlear/dis-cochlear-gen.htm) and includes, at a minimum, an age-specific pneumococcal vaccination.

The surgeon will also review the patient's current medication list and devise a plan for the management of anticoagulant medications prior to the scheduled surgery. The surgeon will also order a preoperative evaluation to ensure that the candidate is able to undergo surgery and the associated anesthetic risk. The preoperative evaluation includes assessment of vital signs and general medical evaluation to identify the presence of health problems which may affect peri- and/or postanesthetic care.

Most implant surgeons also routinely order imaging studies including computed tomography (CT) and/or magnetic resonance imaging (MRI) to determine cochlear patency as well as to rule out cochlear or other temporal bone anomalies that could impact the surgical insertion of the device. Cochlear and temporal bone anomalies, however, are not necessarily contraindicated for cochlear implantation, though it is critical that the surgical team be aware of such issues. High-resolution CT using a temporal bone protocol is typically ordered for all patients having met audiologic criteria for cochlear implantation (Witte et al., 2003). MRI on the other hand, is not generally ordered for adult patients with acquired sensorineural hearing loss, with the exception of those exhibiting audiometric asymmetry.

The surgeon's role also includes careful review of risks associated with cochlear implant surgery and obtaining informed consent for the surgical procedure. It is not within the scope of practice of the audiologist or the speech/language pathologist to initiate the discussion surrounding surgical risk. This is not to say that it is inappropriate to discuss risk with patients should they inquire; however, it is important that we defer thorough discussion and questioning of such matters to the surgeon. For this reason, the medical/surgical consult is typically scheduled *after* the cochlear implant evaluation and workup by the audiologist.

UTILITY OF PREDICTIVE VARIABLES FOR POSTOPERATIVE OUTCOMES

Once a patient is informed that he or she is a candidate for cochlear implantation, in-depth counseling and education is critical. This is directly within the scope of the audiologist and represents a significant portion of the cochlear implant evaluation/workup appointment. Perhaps as important as educating the patient about the function of cochlear implants and what they do, is the focus on what implants *cannot* do, such as restore "normal" hearing and auditory function. In fact, this is a good point in the counseling to review the expectations questionnaire and to reconcile any discrepancies between the patient's expected outcomes and realistic outcomes.

Perhaps the most frequent question that patients ask regarding cochlear implantation is how well they will do, with respect to speech understanding, following surgery. There are a number of potential factors affecting postoperative outcomes including age, audiometric thresholds, preoperative speech perception performance, duration of deafness, integrity of cochlear and neural structures, and etiology.

Age

Given the increased life expectancy of individuals in developed countries and more specifically in the United States (Kochanek, Xu, Murphy, Minino, & Kung, 2011), we will undoubtedly be seeing more elderly individuals for cochlear implant candidacy evaluations. Traditionally, clinicians have proceeded cautiously, recommending implants for elderly individuals with the thought that surgical and audiologic outcomes may be adversely affected by age-related issues as well as that they are associated with lower cost utility. Recently a number of studies have investigated the benefit associated with cochlear implantation in individuals 70 years and older (Carlson et al., 2010; Coelho et al., 2009). These studies have shown no greater anesthetic risk and equivalent degrees of benefit for postoperative speech perception in younger

implant recipients (Buchman, Fucci, & Luxford, 1999; Carlson et al., 2010). In fact, even patients in their tenth decade of life have demonstrated significant postoperative benefit for speech recognition (Carlson et al., 2010). Thus, provided that an individual has been medically cleared for surgery and does not exhibit compromised cognitive status and/or dementia, there are no major concerns about an adult patient's age at implantation in terms of negatively predicting audiologic outcomes.

Role of Audiometric Thresholds

Audiologists and surgeons tend to place considerable emphasis on the audiogram and audiometric thresholds; however, while the audiogram represents a diagnostic measure of an individual's auditory detection or *sensation*, it does not always accurately reflect an individual's auditory function or *perception*. In a study related to hearing aid outcomes, Haplin and Rauch (2009) explained that the audiogram does not represent structural impairments that underlie word recognition ability; hence, audiograms often provide false predictions of hearing aid outcome success. In fact, there are a number of papers reporting data for hearing aid users with audiograms outside the approved candidacy criteria for cochlear implantation who subjectively report and exhibit great difficulty hearing and communicating in real-world situations (Alkaf & Firszt, 2007; Gifford, Dorman, McKarns, & Spahr, 2007; Gifford, Dorman, Shallop, & Sydlowski, 2010; Novak, Black, & Koch, 2007).

Despite the fact that similar audiograms do not necessarily yield similar speech perception performance, it may still seem intuitive that better preoperative audiometric thresholds would yield higher levels of postoperative performance, but this is not the case. In fact, few studies have demonstrated a significant correlation between preoperative audiometric thresholds and postoperative speech perception performance. This is true for both the ear to be implanted (e.g., Battmer, Gupta, Allum-Mecklenburg, & Lenarz, 1995; Blamey et al., 1992; Gantz et al.,1988; Gantz, Woodworth, Knutson, Abbas, & Tyler, 1993; Waltzman, Fisher, Niparko, & Cohen, 1995) as well as the nonimplanted ear (Ching, Incerti, & Hill, 2004; Ching,

Psarros, Hill, Dillon, & Incerti, 2001; Gifford et al., 2007; Potts, Skinner, Litovsky, Strube, & Kuk, 2009; also see Morera et al., 2005). This finding is contrary to both clinical intuition and the long-standing belief that a higher proportion of surviving spiral ganglion cells would likely yield higher levels of postoperative speech recognition. In fact, histopathology data from human temporal bones of individuals who had been cochlear implant recipients suggests that there is no correlation between spiral ganglion cell survival and postoperative speech perception performance (Fayad & Linthicum, 2006; Gassner, Shallop, & Driscoll, 2005; Nadol et al., 2001).

Role of Preoperative Speech Perception and Duration of Deafness

As described above, we as clinicians must challenge ourselves to think "beyond the audiogram" and treat the patient's overall auditory profile and functional performance. In this light, one may hypothesize that higher levels of preoperative speech perception performance would yield higher levels of postoperative performance, but this is not necessarily the case.

In one of the most comprehensive statistical analyses of predictive variables for cochlear implantation, Rubinstein, Parkinson, Tyler, & Gantz (1999) examined a number of potential variables affecting postoperative speech recognition including preoperative sentence-recognition scores, preoperative audiometric thresholds, duration of deafness prior to implantation, and age. Despite the array of factors analyzed in the model, Rubinstein and colleagues found that that duration of deafness and preoperative sentence scores of subjects were consistently found to be the two most significant predictors of postoperative hearing outcomes when factored together in multivariate analysis. The extremes of the function, however, dominate the correlation (Rubinstein et al., 1999). For the comparison of pre-implant sentence recognition with post-implant word recognition, had the pre-implant scores at 0% been removed from the analysis, no correlation would exist (Figure 2–5A). The reason that such a consideration is valid is that those patients scoring 0% preoperatively on CID sentences scored anywhere from 0 to 70% correct for word recognition postoperatively. In a similar vein, examining duration of deafness with postoperative word recognition, had the scores for patients with greater than

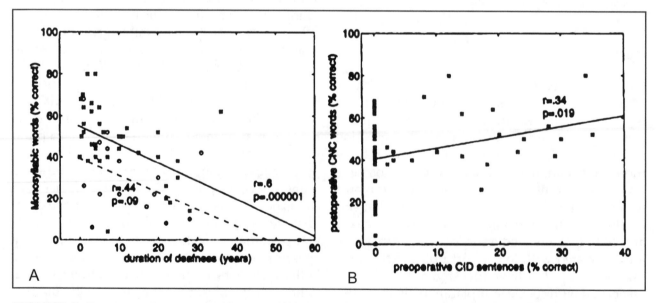

FIGURE 2–5. Shown here is a figure that originally appeared in a classic paper by Rubinstein and colleagues (1999). Correlations are drawn between duration of deafness and postoperative monosyllabic word recognition (*A*) as well as preoperative sentence recognition performance and postoperative word recognition performance (*B*). Reprinted with permission.

20 years of duration of deafness been removed, no correlation would exist (Figure 2–5B). Similar findings have been reported by more recent analyses of patient variables and associated post-operative predictive power (Friedland, Venick, & Niparko, 2003; Leung et al., 2005; Roditi, Poissant, Bero, & Lee, 2009); thus, for a large proportion of cochlear implant candidates—those with shorter durations of deafness and scoring above 0% correct preoperatively—there are currently no definitive predictive variables for postoperative speech recognition.

Integrity of Cochlear and Neural Structures

Cochlear and neural anomalies are generally considered to be most applicable to counseling for pediatric patients; however, there are instances of adult cochlear anomalies and/or auditory neuropathy that are uncovered during the cochlear implant workup process.

Any structural irregularity involving the bony labyrinth, cochlear lumen, or internal auditory canal has the potential to affect postoperative outcomes. Some common structural abnormalities that one might expect to uncover in the adult population include Mondini dysplasia, enlarged vestibular aqueduct, and atretic internal auditory canal. All of these diagnoses would be observed via CT imaging and would thus be diagnosed prior to implantation for adult candidates.

Another issue that can affect postoperative performance is auditory neuropathy. This can be a true neuropathy of the auditory branch of cranial nerve VIII, which is typically associated with other peripheral neuropathies, or an auditory neuropathy spectrum disorder (ANSD) as typically associated with pediatric diagnoses. There have been a number of reported cases of adult-onset ANSD (e.g., Berlin et al., 2010; Kumar & Jayaram, 2005; Prieve, Gorga, & Neely, 1991; Shivashankar, Satishchandra, Shaskikala, & Gore, 2003; Stuart & Mills, 2009). The underlying mechanism for late- or adult-onset ANSD is not well understood. The general profile of ANSD would include variable levels of audiometric thresholds, poorer-than-expected speech recognition, acoustic

reflex thresholds absent in approximately 90% of cases, presence of otoacoustic emissions that are incongruent with the audiogram, and presence of cochlear microphonic with either absent or abnormal auditory brainstem response (e.g., Berlin, Hood, Cecola, Jackson, & Szabo, 1993; Berlin et al, 2010; Berlin et al., 2005; Starr et al., 1996).

A true neuropathy of the auditory nerve is important to diagnose prior to considering cochlear implantation, because it would significantly affect outcomes. The word neuropathy refers to nerve damage; thus, cochlear implantation would be contraindicated for a true case of auditory neuropathy for which there is compromised integrity of the auditory nerve. The reason is that intracochlear electrical stimulation targeting spiral ganglion cells in the modiolus would be peripheral to the site of lesion, and hence, a cochlear implant would not be effective in restoring hearing. True cases of auditory neuropathy often accompany other peripheral neuropathies and include numbness, tingling, and burning of the external ear, face, lips, tongue, and extremities. Should a patient present with these symptoms and is not currently under the care of a neurologist, a referral should be made. Care should be exercised in recommending cochlear implantation for patients presenting with these symptoms because it can be difficult, if not impossible, to distinguish between ANSD and a true case of auditory neuropathy, the latter of which would expectedly yield poor outcomes with cochlear implantation.

Etiology

The etiology of hearing loss for the majority of adult patients seen in an audiology clinic is largely unknown. Consequently, there is generally no concern about etiology affecting counseling for postoperative outcomes. There are, however, some etiologies that are known to potentially affect postoperative outcomes seen with adult cochlear implant recipients.

Meningitis

Although the incidence of bacterial meningitis is lower in adults than in children, it remains a leading cause of acquired sensorineural hearing loss in adults. Epidemiologic studies have reported that the incidence of bacterial meningitis exhibits a twofold increase with age from the range of 18–34 years to the over-65-years population with the mean adult incidence being in the range of 1.3–1.5 cases per 100,000 (Thigpen et al., 2011). The cause of hearing loss associated with bacterial meningitis is typically related to the development of labyrinthitis, loss of hair cells, spiral ganglion cell degeneration, and cochlear ossification (Lu & Schuknecht, 1994; Nadol & Hsu, 1991). It is specifically the ossification and degeneration of spiral ganglion cells that can result in bony obliteration of the cochlea, loss of auditory function, and hence, poorer postoperative outcomes.

Depending on the degree of ossification, it is possible that the surgeon may not be able to achieve a full insertion of the electrode array; thus, the patient may have a restricted number of electrodes that can be stimulated. Furthermore, it is possible that with a shallow electrode insertion depth and spiral ganglion cell degeneration, those intracochlear electrodes may not yield much, if any, auditory stimulation. Reports of postoperative outcomes following meningitis are variable and have been reported as being significantly poorer than that of the typical adult cochlear implant recipient (Battmer et al., 1995; Philippon, Bergeron, Ferron, & Bussieres, 2010; Waltzman et al., 1995). Though this certainly does not apply for all cases of meningitis, it remains an important counseling point for individuals with this diagnosis.

Otosclerosis

The pathogenesis of otosclerosis includes temporal bone dysplasia, which is often referred to as an otospongiotic or bony growth that can pervade the bony labyrinth. Cochlear implantation for patients with otosclerosis is routinely performed and is typically associated with excellent postoperative outcomes (Marshall et al., 2005; Quaranta et al., 2005; Sainz, García-Valdecasas, Garófano, & Ballesteros, 2007). Due to the progression of the underlying disease process, however, there are some factors to consider with regard to postoperative outcomes. The continued progression of bony

growth is known to affect the intracochlear transmission of the electrical signal which can result in variable thresholds for stimulation, charge, and facial nerve stimulation due to current shunting (Carlson et al., 2011; Sainz, Garcia-Valdecasas, & Ballesteros 2009). Consequently, it is often the case that the number of usable electrodes decreases and/or varies over time. Variation in the number of usable electrodes has the potential to impact patient performance, overall auditory perception, and sound quality; thus, these issues should be addressed in preoperative counseling during the cochlear implant evaluation/workup appointment.

CONCLUSION

The opening of this chapter stated that determining cochlear implant candidacy is not a straightforward process. The determination of cochlear implant candidacy is truly a *process* that is accomplished via the collective teamwork of a multidisciplinary group of professionals. Many patients and their families are astonished at the intricacies involved in a cochlear implant workup evaluation. Given the expansion of adult cochlear implant criteria, widespread insurance coverage for bilateral implantation (see Chapters 5 and 9), and increased incidence of hearing preservation (see Chapters 5 and 9) with cochlear implantation, the implant selection process will continue to evolve. Furthermore, we will likely see an even greater role for pre- and postoperative counseling as cochlear implant criteria expand allowing greater numbers of individuals with various degrees of hearing loss and underlying etiologies to take advantage of this technology.

REFERENCES

Abrams, T. E., Barnett, M. J., Hoth, A., Schultz, S., & Kaboli, P. J. (2006). The relationship between hearing impairment and depression in older veterans. *Journal of the American Geriatric Society, 54,* 1475–1477.

Alkaf, F. M., & Firszt, J. B. (2007). Speech recognition in quiet and noise in borderline cochlear implant candidates. *Journal of the American Academy of Audiology, 18*(10), 872–882.

ANSI. (1999, R2003). *Maximum permissible ambient noise levels for audiometric test rooms.* New York, NY: American National Standards Institute, S3.1-1999.

Balkany, T., Hodges, A., Menapace, C., Hazard, L., Driscoll, C., Gantz, B., . . . Payne, S. (2007). Nucleus Freedom North American clinical trial. *Otolaryngology—Head and Neck Surgery, 136,* 757–762.

Battmer, R. D., Gupta, S. P., Allum-Mecklenburg, D. J., & Lenarz, T. (1995). Factors influencing cochlear implant perceptual performance in 132 adults. In G. M. Clark, & R. S. C. Cowan (Eds.), International Cochlear Implant, Speech and Hearing Symposium, Melbourne 1994. *Annals of Otology, Rhinology and Laryngology* (Suppl. 166), 185–187.

Berlin, C. I., Hood, L. J., Cecola, R. P., Jackson, D. F., & Szabo, P. (1993). Does Type I afferent neuron dysfunction reveal itself through lack of efferent suppression? *Hearing Research, 65,* 40–50.

Berlin, C.I., Hood, L. J., Morlet, T., Wilensky, D., Li, L., Mattingly, K. R., Taylor-Jeanfreau, J., . . . Frisch, S. A. (2010). Multi-site diagnosis and management of 260 patients with auditory neuropathy/dys-synchrony (auditory neuropathy spectrum disorder). *International Journal of Audiology, 49,* 30–43.

Berlin, C. I., Hood, L. J., Mortlet, T., Wilensky, D., St. John, P., Montgomery, E., & Thibodaux, M. (2005). Absent or elevated middle ear muscle reflexes in the presence of normal otoacoustic emissions: A universal finding in 136 cases of auditory neuropathy/dyssynchrony. *Journal of American Academy of Audiology, 16,* 546–553.

Blamey, P. J., Pyman, B. C., Gordon, M., Clark, G. M., Brown, A. M., Dowell, R. C., & Hollow, R. D. (1992). Factors predicting postoperative sentence scores in postlinguistically deaf adult cochlear implant patients. *Annals of Otology Rhinology and Laryngology, 101,* 342–348.

Buchman, C. A., Fucci, M. J., & Luxford, W. M. (1999). Cochlear implants in the geriatric population: Benefits outweigh risks. *Ear, Nose & Throat Journal, 78,* 489–494.

Busen, J., & McCarthy, P. (2010). *Probe-microphone measurements: Commonly used or neglected?* Presented at AudiologyNOW!, San Diego, CA.

Carhart, R. L. (1949). Monitored live-voice as a test of auditory acuity. *Journal of the Acoustical Society of America, 17,* 339–349.

Carlson, M. L., Driscoll, C. L. W., Gifford, R. H., Service, G. J., Tombers, N. M., Hughes-Borst, B. J., . . . Beatty, C. W. (2011). Implications of minimizing trauma during conventional cochlear implantation. *Otology & Neurotology, 32,* 962–968.

Carlson, M. L., Breen, J. T., Gifford, R. H., Driscoll, C. L. W., Neff, B. A., Beatty, C. W., . . . Olund, A. P. (2010). Cochlear implantation in the octogenarian and nonagenarian. *Otology & Neurotology, 31,* 1343–1349.

Centers for Medicare & Medicaid Services (CMS). (2005). *National coverage determination (NCD) for cochlear implantation (50.3).* Publication No. 100-3. Available at http://www.cms.gov/medicare-coverage-database/details/ncd-details.aspx?NCDId=245&ncdver=2&bc=BAABAAAAAAAA&

Ching, T. Y., Incerti, P., & Hill, M. (2004). Binaural benefits for adults who use hearing aids and cochlear implants in the opposite ears. *Ear and Hearing, 25,* 9–21.

Ching, T. Y., Psarros, C., Hill, M. Dillon, H., & Incerti, P. (2001). Should children who use cochlear implants wear hearing aids in the opposite ear? *Ear and Hearing, 22,* 365–380.

Cochlear Corporation. (2003). *Pre and post-operative evaluation manual for Nucleus® cochlear implant systems.* FUZ139 ISS3, Oct 2003.

Coelho, D. H., Yeh, J., Kim, J. T., & Lalwani, A. K. (2009). Cochlear implantation is associated with minimal anesthetic risk in the elderly. *Laryngoscope, 119,* 355–358.

Cox, R. M., & Alexander, G. C. (1995). The abbreviated profile of hearing aid benefit. *Ear and Hearing, 16,* 176–186.

Deltenre, P., Mansbach, A. L., Bozet, C., Christiaens, F., Barthelemy, P., Paulissen, D., & Renglet, T. (1999). Auditory neuropathy with preserved cochlear microphonics and secondary loss of otoacoustic emissions. *Audiology, 38,* 187–195.

Dillon, H., James, A., & Ginis, J. (1997). The Client Oriented Scale of Improvement (COSI) and its relationship to several other measures of benefit and satisfaction provided by hearing aids. *Journal of the American Academy of Audiology, 8,* 27–43.

Dirks, D. D., Morgan, D. E., & Wilson, R. H. (1976). Experimental audiology. In C. A. Smith & J. A. Vernon (Eds.), *Handbook of auditory and vestibular research methods* (pp. 517–531). Springfield, IL: Charles C Thomas.

Fabry, D., Firszt, J. B., Gifford, R. H., Holden, L. K., & Koch, D. (2009). Evaluating speech perception benefit in adult cochlear implant recipients. *Audiology Today, 21,* 37–42.

Fayad, J. N., & Linthicum, F. H. (2006). Multichannel cochlear implants: relation of histopathology to performance. *Laryngoscope, 116,* 1310–1320.

FDA NCT01066780. (2010). ClearVoice sound-processing strategy for AB HiRes 120 cochlear implant users. Food and Drug Administration clinical trial. Valencia, CA: Advanced Bionics.

Firszt, J. B., Holden, L. K., Skinner, M. W., Tobey, E. A., Peterson, A., Gaggl, W., . . . Wackym, P. A. (2004). Recognition of speech presented at soft to loud levels by adult cochlear implant recipients of three cochlear implant systems. *Ear and Hearing, 25*(4), 375–387.

Friedland, D. R., Venick, H. S., & Niparko, J. K. (2003). Choice of ear for cochlear implantation: The effect of history and residual hearing on predicted post-operative performance. *Otology & Neurotology, 24*, 582–589.

Furlong, W. J., Feeny, D. H., Torrance, G. W., & Barr, R. D. (2001). The Health Utilities Index (HUI) system for assessing health-related quality of life in clinical studies. *Annals of Medicine, 33*, 375–384.

Gantz, B. J., Hansen, M. R., Turner, C. W., Oleson, J. J., Reiss, L. A., & Parkinson, A. J. (2009). Hybrid 10 clinical trial: Preliminary results. *Audiology & Neurotology, 14*(Suppl. 1), 32–38.

Gantz, B. J., Tyler, R. S., Knutson, J. F., Woodworth, G., Abbas, P., McCabe, B. F., . . . Kuk, F. (1988). Evaluation of five different cochlear implant designs: Audiologic assessment and predictors of performance. *Laryngoscope, 98*, 1100–1106.

Gantz, B. J., Woodworth, G. G., Knutson, J. F., Abbas, P. J., & Tyler, R. S. (1993). Multivariate predictors of audiological success with multichannel cochlear implants. *Annals of Otology, Rhinology, and Laryngology, 102*, 909–916.

Gassner, H. G., Shallop, J. K., & Driscoll, C. L. W. (2005). Long-term clinical course and temporal bone histology after cochlear implantation. *Cochlear Implants International, 6*, 67–78.

Gatehouse, S. (1999). A self-report outcome measure for the evaluation of hearing aid fittings and services. *Health Bulletin, 57*, 424–436.

Gifford, R. H., Dorman, M. F., McKarns, S. A., & Spahr, A. (2007). Combined electric and contralateral acoustic hearing: Word and sentence recognition with bimodal hearing. *Journal of Speech and Language Hearing Research, 50*(4), 835–843.

Gifford, R. H., Dorman, M. F., Shallop, J. K., & Sydlowski, S. (2010). Evidence for the expansion of adult cochlear implant candidacy. *Ear and Hearing, 31*(2), 186–194.

Gifford, R., Shallop, J. K., & Peterson A. M. (2008). Speech recognition materials and ceiling effects: Considerations for cochlear implant programs. *Audiology & Neurotology, 13*, 193–205.

Gopinath, B., Wang, J. J., Schneider, J., Burlutsky, G., Snowdon, J., McMahon, C. M., . . . Mitchell, P. (2009). Depressive symptoms in older adults with hearing impairments: the Blue Mountains Study. *Journal of American Geriatric Society, 57*(7), 1306–1308.

Gstoettner, W. K., van de Heyning, P., O'Connor, A. F., Morera, C., Sainz, M., Vermeire, K., . . . Adunka, O. F. (2008). Electric acoustic stimulation of the auditory system: Results of a multi-centre investigation. *Acta Oto-Laryngologica, 128*, 968–975.

Haplin, C., & Rauch, S. D. (2009). Hearing aids and cochlear damage: The case against fitting the pure tone audiogram. *Otolaryngology Head and Neck Surgery, 140*, 629–632.

Hinderink, J. B., Krabbe, P. F. M., & Broek, P. V. D. (2000). Development and application of a health-related quality-of-life instrument for adults with cochlear implants: The Nijmegen Cochlear Implant Questionnaire. *Otolaryngology—Head and Neck Surgery, 123*, 756–765.

Killion, M., Niquette, P., Revit, L., & Skinner, M. (2001). Quick SIN and BKB-SIN: Two new speech-in-noise tests permitting SNR-50 estimates in 1 to 2 min (A). *Journal of the Acoustical Society of America, 109*(5), 2502–2512.

Knutson, J. F., Johnson, A., & Murray, K. T. (2006). Social and emotional characteristics of adults seeking a cochlear implant and their spouses. *British Journal of Health Psychology, 11*(Pt. 2), 279–292.

Knutson, J. F., Murray, K. T., Husarek, S., Westerhouse, K., Woodworth, G. Gantz, B. J., & Tyler, R. S. (1998). Psychological change over 54 months of cochlear implant use. *Ear and Hearing, 19*, 191–201.

Knutson, J. F., Schartz, H. A., Gantz, B. J., Tyler, R. S., Hinrichs, J. V., & Woodworth, G. (1991). Psychological change following 18 months of cochlear implant use. *Annals of Otology, Rhinology, and Laryngology, 100*, 877–882.

Kochanek, K. D., Xu, J., Murphy, S. L., Minino, A. M., & Kung, H. C. (2011). Deaths: Preliminary data for 2009. *National Vital Statistics Reports, 59*(4), 1–51.

Kumar, A. U., & Jayaram, M. (2005). Auditory processing in individuals with auditory neuropathy. *Behavioral Brain Function, 1*, 1–21.

Leung, J., Wang, N. Y., Yeagle, J. D., Chinnici, J., Bowditch, S., Francis, H. W., & Niparko, J. K. (2005). Predictive models for cochlear implantation in elderly candidates. *Archives of Otolaryngology-Head & Neck Surgery, 131*, 1049–1054.

Lu, C. B., & Schuknecht, H. F. (1994). Pathology of prelingual profound deafness. *American Journal of Otology, 15*, 74–85.

Marshall, A. H., Fanning, N., Symons, S., Shipp, D., Chen, J. M., & Nedzelski, J. M. (2005). Cochlear implantation in cochlear otosclerosis. *Laryngoscope, 115*, 1728Y33.

Martin, F. N., Champlin, C., & Chambers, J. A. (1998). Seventh survey of audiometric practices in the United States. *Journal of the American Academy of Audiology, 9*(2), 95–104.

Medwetsky, L., Sanderson, D., & Young, D. (1999). A national survey of audiology clinical practices, part 1. *Hearing Review, 6*(11), 24–32.

Morera, C., Manrique, M., Ramos, A., Garcia-Ibanez, L., Cavalle, L., Huarte, A., . . . Estrada, E. (2005). Advantages of binaural hearing provided through bimodal stimulation via a cochlear implant and a conventional hearing aid: A 6-month comparative study. *Acta Otolaryngologica, 125*, 596–606.

Nachtegaal, J., Smit, J. H., Smits, C., Bezemer, P. D., van Beek, J. H., Festen, J. M., & Kramer, S. E. (2009). The association between hearing status and psychosocial health before the age of 70 years: Results from an Internet-based national survey on hearing. *Ear and Hearing, 30*(3), 302–312.

Nadol, J. B., & Hsu, W. (1991). Histopathologic correlation of spiral ganglion. *Annals of Otology, Rhinology, and Laryngology, 100*, 712–716.

Nadol, J. B., Shiao, J. Y., Burgess, B. J., Ketten, D. R., Eddington, D. K., Gantz, B. J., . . . Shallop, J. K. (2001). Histopathology of cochlear implants in humans. *Annals of Otology, Rhinology, and Laryngology, 110*, 883–891.

Newman, C. W., Weinstein, B. E., Jacobson, G. P., & Hug, G. A. (1990). The Hearing Handicap Inventory for Adults: psychometric adequacy and audiometric correlates. *Ear and Hearing, 11*, 430–433.

Nilsson, M., Soli, S., & Sullivan, J. (1994). Development of the Hearing in Noise test for the measurement of speech reception thresholds in quiet and in noise. *Journal of the Acoustical Society of America, 95*, 1085–1099.

Nilsson, M. J., McCaw, V. M., & Soli, S. (1996). *Minimum speech test battery for adult cochlear implant users: User manual.* Los Angeles, CA: House Ear Institute.

Novak, M. A., Black, J. M., & Koch, D. B. (2007). Standard cochlear implantation of adults with residual low-frequency hearing: Implications for combined electro-acoustic stimulation. *Otology & Neurotology, 28*(5), 609–614.

Olze, H., Szczepek, A. J., Haupt, H., Förster, U., Zirke, N., Gräbel, S., & Mazurek, B. (2011). Cochlear implantation has a positive influence on quality of life, tinnitus, and psychological comorbidity. *Laryngoscope, 121*(10), 2220–2227.

Patrick, D. L., & Erickson, P. (1993). *Health status and health policy: Quality of life in health care evaluation and resource allocation.* New York, NY: Oxford University Press.

Pearsons, K. S., Bennett, R. L., & Fidell, S. (1977). *Speech levels in various noise environments* (Report No. EPA-600/1-77-025). Washington, DC: U.S. Environmental Protection Agency.

Peterson, G. E., & Lehiste, I. (1962). Revised CNC lists for auditory tests. *Journal of Speech and Hearing Disorders, 27*, 62–72.

Philippon, D., Bergeron, F., Ferron, P., & Bussieres, R. (2010). Cochlear implantation in postmeningitic deafness. *Otology & Neurotology, 31*, 83–87.

Poissant, S. F., Beaudoin, F., Huang, J., Brodsky, J., & Lee, D. J. (2008). Impact of cochlear implantation on speech understanding, depression, and loneliness in the elderly. *Journal of Otolaryngology — Head and Neck Surgery, 37*(4), 488–494.

Potts, L. G., Skinner, M. W., Litovsky, R. A., Strube, M. J., & Kuk, F. (2009). Recognition and localization of speech by adult cochlear implant recipients wearing a digital hearing aid in the nonimplanted ear (bimodal hearing). *Journal of the American Academy of Audiology, 20*, 353–373.

Prieve, B. A., Gorga, M. P., & Neely, S. T. (1991). Otoacoustic emissions in an adult with severe hearing loss. *Journal of Speech Language and Hearing Research, 34*, 379–385.

Quaranta, N., Bartoli, R., Lopriore, A., Fernandez-Vega, S., Giagnotti, F., & Quaranta, F. (2005). Cochlear implantation in otosclerosis. *Otology & Neurotology, 26*, 983–987.

Raffin, M. J. M., & Thornton, A. R. (1980). Confidence levels for differences between speech-discrimination scores: A research note. *Journal of Speech and Hearing Research, 23*, 5–18.

Robinson, K., Gatehouse, S., & Browning, G. G. (1996). Measuring patient benefit from otorhinolaryngological surgery and therapy. *Annals of Otology, Rhinology, and Laryngology, 105*, 415–422.

Roditi, R. E., Poissant, S. F., Bero, E. M., & Lee, D. J. (2009). A predictive model of cochlear implant performance in postlingually deafened adults. *Otology & Neurotology, 30*, 449–454.

Roeser, R., & Clark, J. (2008). Live voice speech recognition audiometry: Stop the madness. *Audiology Today, 20*, 32–33.

Rubinstein, J. T., Parkinson, W. S., Tyler, R. S., & Gantz, B. J. (1999). Residual speech recognition and cochlear implant performance: Effects of implantation criteria. *American Journal of Otology, 20*(4), 445–452.

Sainz, M., Garcia-Valdecasas, J., & Ballesteros, J. M. (2009). Complications and pitfalls of cochlear implantation in otosclerosis: A 6-year follow-up cohort study. *Otology & Neurotology, 30*, 1044–1048.

Sainz, M., García-Valdecasas, J., Garófano M., & Ballesteros, J. M. (2007). Otosclerosis: Mid-term results of cochlear implantation. *Audiology & Neurotology, 12,* 401–406.

Shivashankar, N., Satishchandra, P., Shashikala, H. R., & Gore, M. (2003). Primary auditory neuropathy: An enigma. *Acta Neurologica Scandinavica, 108,* 130–135.

Skarzynski, H., Lorens, A., Piotrowska, A., & Anderson, I. (2006). Partial deafness cochlear implantation provides benefit to a new population of individuals with hearing loss. *Acta Oto-Laryngologica, 126,* 934–940.

Skinner, M. W., Holden, L. K., Holden, T. A., Demorest, M. E., & Fourakis, M. S. (1997). Speech recognition at simulated soft, conversational, and raised-to-loud vocal efforts by adults with cochlear implants. *Journal of the Acoustical Society of America, 101*(6), 3766–3782.

Spahr, A. J., Dorman, M. F., Litvak, L. L., Van Wie, S., Gifford, R. H., Loizou, P. C., . . . Cook, S. (2012). Development and validation of the AzBio sentence lists. *Ear and Hearing, 33,* 112–117.

Starr, A., Picton, T. W., Sininger, Y., Hood, L. J., & Berlin, C. I. (1996). Auditory neuropathy. *Brain, 119,* 741–753.

Stuart, A., & Mills, K. N. (2009). Late-onset unilateral auditory neuropathy/dysynchrony: A case study. *Journal of the American Academy of Audiology, 20,* 172–179.

Thigpen, M. C., Whitney, C. G., Messonnier, N. E., Zell, E. R., Lynfield, R., Hadler, J. L., . . . Schuchat, A., for the Emerging Infections Programs Network. (2011). Bacterial meningitis in the United States, 1998–2007. *New England Journal of Medicine, 26, 364*(21), 2016–2025.

Tucker, M. A. (2001). *A time study of audiological practice patterns and the impact of reimbursement changes from third party payers.* Unpublished thesis, University of South Florida, Tampa, FL.

Valente, M., Abrams, H., Benson, D., Chisolm, T., Citron, D., Hampton, D., . . . Sweetow, R. (2006). Guidelines for the audiologic management of adult hearing impairment. *Audiology Today, 18*(5), 1–44.

Ventry, I. M., & Weinstein, B. E. (1982). The Hearing Handicap Inventory for the Elderly: A new tool. *Ear and Hearing, 3,* 128–134.

Wackym, P. A., Runge-Samuelson, C. L., Firszt, J. B., Alkaf, F. M., & Burg, L. S. (2007). More challenging speech perception tasks demonstrate binaural benefit in bilateral cochlear implant users. *Ear and Hearing, 28,* 80S–85S.

Waltzman, S. B., Fisher, S. G., Niparko, J. K., & Cohen, N. L. (1995). Predictors of postoperative performance with cochlear implants. *Annals of Otology, Rhinology, and Laryngology Supplement, 165,* 15–18.

Witte, R. J., Lane, J. I., Driscoll, C. L., Lundy, L. B., Bernstein, M. A., Kotsenas, A. L., & Kocharian, A. (2003). Pediatric and adult cochlear implantation. *Radiographics, 23*(5), 1185–1200.

3

Pediatric Cochlear Implant Candidate Selection

René H. Gifford

INTRODUCTION

As mentioned in Chapter 2, determining cochlear implant candidacy is not necessarily a straightforward process. This is particularly true when assessing candidacy for infants and children. Pediatric cochlear implant criteria have continued to evolve since the Food and Drug Administration (FDA) first approved multichannel cochlear implants for children in June 1990. For children, candidacy criteria vary with age, etiology, as well as across the different manufacturers. Furthermore, there are a number of auditory-related milestones for which, even if they are not met, implant candidacy may be determined regardless of whether the child meets the typical candidate profile.

There are a number of aspects requiring careful consideration in the process of pediatric cochlear implant candidate selection. Many of these aspects are related to the audiologic evaluation including audiometric and speech recognition testing; others are related to speech and language development. There are also medical, radiologic, and psychological issues requiring consideration.

This chapter discusses pediatric cochlear implant candidate selection including aspects to be considered from the perspective of the audiologist, speech/language pathologist, social worker and/or psychologist, as well as the medical/surgical team. The chapter also describes the elements of cochlear implant candidate selection for children with hearing loss as it stands today as well as discusses those elements that, as a field, we may want to consider in the evaluation process.

AUDIOLOGIC EVALUATION

Assessment of Hearing Status

As with adult candidacy evaluations, virtually all pediatric cochlear implant evaluations begin in the audiology clinic. The cochlear implant evaluation is ordinarily preceded by numerous appointments in the diagnostic audiology clinic for behavioral hearing testing as well as objective estimates of auditory function including otoacoustic emissions and auditory brainstem response. The pediatric cochlear implant evaluation process does not involve the initial diagnosis of a severe-to-profound hearing loss as children and their families present to the evaluation with a confirmed diagnosis and hearing aid experience; thus, the family arrives at the appointment with knowledge and at least partial acceptance of the diagnosis. This generally helps facilitate discussion about cochlear implants without the presence of a raw emotional component that is known to accompany new diagnoses. For those audiologists engaging in all aspects of pediatric audiologic care, a patient and family will be followed from initial diagnosis to hearing aid fittings, follow-up, and assessment of auditory progress through determination of candidacy. Given the demand for highly skilled pediatric cochlear implant audiologists, it is generally not the case that a single provider is involved in all previous diagnostic- and amplification-related appointments.

Despite the fact that most families present to the first implant evaluation with prior audiograms and objective estimates of auditory function, it is recommended that comprehensive audiometric testing be completed. This is an obvious opportunity to gain additional ear-specific pure-tone and speech awareness information particularly for frequencies that prior audiograms may have been lacking. It is also appropriate to complete tympanograms and, at a minimum, ipsilateral acoustic reflex testing. Given that multiple assessments of behavioral hearing status are recommended prior to finalizing candidate selection, it is generally the case that a child is not seen by the cochlear implant team for assessment at least until 6 months age, which is generally the age at which reliable behavioral assessment of hearing can be completed; thus, the earliest implant evaluation/workup appointments involve visual reinforcement audiometry and/or behavioral observation audiometry. This task becomes more complicated for the assessment of children with concomitant diagnoses that may delay sitting up, independent head and neck control, and more global developmental and/or cognitive abilities.

Otoacoustic emissions (OAEs) provide valuable information for the cochlear implant evaluation. Although most newborn hearing screening programs in well-baby nurseries utilize OAEs as a first-pass screening tool (e.g., NIH, 1993; White et al., 2005; Gravel et al., 2005; JCIH, 2007), not all children will have had this completed. Virtually every cochlear implant audiologist has at least one story about a patient presenting for an evaluation who is diagnosed with auditory neuropathy spectrum disorder (ANSD) *after* the cochlear implant evaluation appointment. Although ANSD does not preclude a patient from cochlear implantation (e.g., Shallop et al., 2001; Peterson et al., 2003; Rance & Barker, 2008; Teagle et al., 2010; Breneman et al., 2012), it is important to have an accurate diagnosis in place as well as to explore all possible habilitative options prior to pursuing surgical intervention.

Cochlear Implant Criteria: Audiometric Thresholds

Cochlear implant criteria, with respect to audiometric thresholds, differ across implant manufacturers. For pediatric candidacy, there is an additional element of age-specific audiometric criteria. For children age 12–24 months, the current criteria specify bilateral *profound* sensorineural hearing loss (Cochlear Americas package insert, Advanced Bionics package insert, MED-EL package insert). This is not to imply that children with less severe hearing losses would not benefit from cochlear implantation. Rather, the historical concern has been that obtaining behavioral thresholds for the youngest children was more difficult than for older children; hence, the criteria were most stringent for the youngest candidates. This concern may not be as valid today given the audiologic checks and balances that are at our disposal for both behavioral assessments of hearing and objective/physiologic estimates of auditory function. In fact, this is also an argument for lowering the FDA-approved age for cochlear implantation from 12 months to slightly younger—perhaps in the 6- to 9-month range (e.g., Cosetti & Roland, 2010; Kim, Jeong, Lee, & Kim, 2010). Research has demonstrated higher levels of word and language acquisition (Bergeson, Houston, & Miyamoto, 2010; Houston, Stewart, Moberly, Hollich, & Miyamoto, 2010; Niparko et al., 2010; Moog & Geers, 2010), speech perception (Tajudeen et al., 2010), speech production intelligibility (Habib, Waltzman, Tajudeen, & Svirsky., 2010), and vocabulary development (Hayes, Geers, Treiman, & Moog.2009; Houston & Miyamoto, 2010; Tomblin et al., 2005) for children implanted early—even for those implanted under 12 months of age compared with those in the second year of life.

There are a number of developmental changes occurring within the first year of life that may be missed for the infant with severe-to-profound hearing loss. This is true even for those infants with appropriately fitted hearing aids given that the audibility may be insufficient to allow for consistent auditory access to spoken language. Word segmentation, which is the process of dividing connected discourse into meaningful units, such as individual words, has been shown to develop rapidly between 7.5 and 10.5 months (e.g., Jusczyk, 2002). By 8 months of age, babies have the capacity for long-term storage of new words, which is an important prerequisite for auditory-based language learning (Jusczyk & Hohne, 1997; Houston & Jusczyk, 2003). Thus the infant with severe-to-profound sensorineural hearing loss, for whom aided audibility is limited, is missing out on the development of these critical auditory-based, language-learning opportunities. The reality is that if a child is not making auditory progress with full-time use of appropriately fitted hearing aids and compliance with the recommended intervention and therapy schedule, that child meets cochlear implant "candidacy" based on the professional clinical judgment of the cochlear implant team (see Chapter 1).

For children over 2 years of age, the audiometric criteria for implantation with a Nucleus device are more lenient, including bilateral severe-to-profound sensorineural hearing loss, allowing for slightly more residual acoustic hearing for candidacy qualification (Cochlear Americas package insert). Both Advanced Bionics and MED-EL, however, continue to list bilateral profound sensorineural hearing loss in the labeled indications for children over 2 years of age. Nevertheless, if a child has moderate-to-profound sensorineural hearing loss and is not making auditory progress

with appropriately fitted hearing aids and intervention, the cochlear implant team has the professional clinical judgment to determine candidacy (see Chapter 1).

SPEECH-RECOGNITION TESTING

Recorded Materials

A central component of pediatric cochlear implant evaluations for older children involves the behavioral assessment of speech recognition abilities. Many children with hearing loss rely heavily on visual cues such as lip reading and more global nonverbal communication; thus, in order to gain an understanding of an individual's auditory-based speech recognition abilities, speech stimuli are presented without visual cues.

As with adult candidacy assessment, the most important aspect surrounding the administration of speech recognition testing for older children involves the use of recorded speech materials. As shown in Chapter 2, Figure 2–1, it is clear that the variability associated with monitored live voice (MLV) presentation does not lend itself well to the assessment of pediatric cochlear implant candidacy. It is important to note, however, that there are some pediatric speech metrics that are not currently available in recorded format. These metrics include Glendonald Auditory Screening Procedure (GASP) words and sentences (Erber, 1982) and the Early Speech Perception (ESP) low verbal pattern perception (Moog & Geers, 1990). These materials, however, are not indicated for use in the determination of implant candidacy and thus do not influence whether or not a child qualifies for implant candidacy. At the time of chapter preparation, Advanced Bionics' package insert of FDA-labeled indications specify administration of the Multisyllabic Lexical Neighborhood Test (MLNT) (Kirk, Pisoni, & Osberger 1995) administered using MLV (70 dB SPL). Given that the MLNT and its monosyllabic equivalent, the Lexical Neighborhood Test (LNT) (Kirk et al., 1995) are available in recorded format, MLV presentation would be contraindicated by best practices for pediatric audiology.

Despite the variability and associated problems with assessing speech recognition via MLV, depending on a child's age and/or global developmental status, MLV may be required to elicit reliable responses. Live voice from a familiar, trusted audiologist is a simpler speech recognition task from that using a recorded speech stimulus. The recorded voice is unfamiliar and often lacks the affect that is found in the speaking style of an individual trained to work with children. It is also for this reason that overly accentuated suprasegmental features of a pediatric audiologist's spoken words along with a slower rate of speech may yield higher levels of speech recognition than that experienced in everyday communicative settings. Furthermore, the test/retest reliability of speech recognition performance obtained via MLV is poorer than that for recorded stimuli (Carhart, 1946; Kruel, Bell, & Nixon, 1969), and thus it is not appropriate for use in cochlear implant candidate selection. Should a child respond only to a familiar voice via MLV and continue to exhibit poor recognition, it is reasonable to determine implant candidacy because speech recognition with standardized, recorded stimuli is either equivalent to or poorer than that obtained via MLV (Roeser & Clark, 2008). (See Chapter 2 for detailed information regarding calibration of recorded stimuli for presentation in the sound field.)

Presentation Level

An important aspect of speech recognition testing for cochlear implant evaluations involves the presentation level of the recorded speech stimuli.

As discussed in Chapter 2, 70 dB SPL is no longer considered an acceptable presentation level for it is not representative of average conversational level speech (Pearsons et al., 1977; Olsen, 1998). Best practices recommendations for adult implant assessments have included the use of recorded speech materials presented at 60 dBA (see Chapter 2) for assessment of speech recognition for pre- as well as post-implant testing; thus, it also follows that the *highest* presentation level for pediatric candidacy assessment would be 60 dBA. There are, however, a number of papers in support of using a lower presentation level for both adults and children given that the average, casual speech levels for children and women range from 50 to 56 dBA (Table 3–1) (Pearson et al., 1977; Olsen, 1998). Given the average levels of speech for different talkers (see Table 3–1), in order to assess speech recognition to gauge a child's understanding of both women and his or her peers, lower presentation levels should also be considered.

Multiple Estimates of Speech Recognition

Unlike candidacy assessment for adult patients, older children fitted with hearing aids may be seen multiple times over several months—this is particularly true for the borderline implant candidate. Multiple visits are required in order to determine whether or not a child is making progress with appropriately fitted hearing aids and intervention. Although there are not currently any recommended guidelines for the frequency of candidacy-based

Table 3–1. Mean speech levels (in dBA) and unweighted sound pressure levels for casual, normal, raised, loud, and shouted speech by men, women, and children in an anechoic chamber*

	Casual	*Normal*	*Raised*	*Loud*	*Shouted*
Women	50 [54] (4)	55 [58] (4)	63 [65] (4)	71 [72] (6)	82 [82] (7)
Men	52 [56] (4)	58 [61] (4)	65 [68] (5)	76 [77] (6)	89 [89] (7)
Children	53 [56] (5)	58 [61] (5)	65 [67] (7)	74 [75] (9)	82 [82] (9)

*Unweighted sound pressure levels are given in brackets and standard deviations are given in parentheses. All values are rounded to the nearest decibel.

Source: From Olsen (1998) and Pearsons et al. (1977)

assessment and the time period over which these assessments should take place, FDA-labeled indications state that a hearing aid trial of at least 6 months should be completed prior to determining candidacy; thus, it is the responsibility of each implant team to determine their own protocol dictating the number of audiologic assessments that should take place over that 6-month period. The obvious exception lies in cases of meningitis for which ossification can limit electrode insertion and outcomes; FDA-labeled criteria currently specify that a shorter hearing aid trial is acceptable and appropriate in such cases. Shorter hearing aid trials are also standard practice in cases of older children who have experienced progressive hearing loss, sudden onset hearing loss, or children who have simply not been making age-appropriate gains in speech and language development with appropriate amplification. The primary concern regarding a compressed hearing aid trial is that the least invasive treatment option be fully considered prior to determination of implant candidacy.

Speech-Recognition Test Materials in Children 3 Years of Age or Less

Current labeled indications for pediatric cochlear implantation do not make reference to closed-set metrics of speech perception as listed here, though this does not mean that these metrics are not valuable instruments in a clinician's toolbox for assessing speech recognition performance and progress prior to determining implant candidacy. Such metrics should be used to assess speech recognition for the youngest patients if for no other reason than to provide a baseline measurement against which preoperative progress with hearing aids and/or postoperative progress can be gauged.

Auditory-skills development for the younger child is usually gauged via auditory questionnaire data, parental report, and speech/language assessment. This is particularly true for the youngest children with severe-to-profound sensorineural hearing loss for whom we expect little progress on auditory skills and auditory/oral language development. The obvious exception to this rule is in the case of younger children with acquired hearing loss and/or progressive hearing loss.

There are a variety of standardized measures of speech recognition that are appropriate for the younger child. Audiologists generally begin with closed-set tests for which a limited set of possible choices are available and a verbal response is not required. One of the most commonly used closed-set tests is the Northwestern University Children's Perception of Speech (NU-CHIPS) (Elliott & Katz, 1980). The NU-CHIPS test contains a picture booklet, each page with four illustrated pictures representing phonetically similar words such as snake, cake, grapes, and sink. The vocabulary level of the NU-CHIPS is in the range of 2.5–5 years. With its four-choice sample, chance performance for NU-CHIPS is 25%.

Slightly more difficult than NU-CHIPS is the Word Identification Picture Intelligibility (WIPI) (Ross and Lehman, 1979) metric. Similar to NU-CHIPS, the WIPI test contains a picture booklet with each page displaying six illustrated pictures representing phonetically similar words such as sled, red, thread, head, bed, and bread. The minimum vocabulary level of the WIPI test is 3–5 years and chance performance is 16.7% correct.

Other computer-based metrics of childhood speech recognition are available which may provide a more interactive, gamelike experience for children growing increasingly tech savvy. The Children's Realistic Intelligibility of Speech Perception (CRISP) and the CRISP Jr. were developed at the University of Wisconsin Madison in the laboratory of Ruth Litovsky, Ph.D.. The CRISP is considered most appropriate for children age 4–7 years. The stimuli include a closed set of 25 spondees and the level of the spondees are varied adaptively to achieve a speech-reception threshold (SRT). The CRISP Jr. (Garadat & Litovsky, 2007) is a variation of the CRISP that is more appropriate for children age 2.5–5 years. Crisp Jr. includes a closed set of 16 words with the names of objects and/or body parts. The CRISP can be administered in a manual scoring method or via computer game interaction with the patient. The speech stimuli can be presented in quiet or in the presence of a background noise originating from the same source as the target or from a separate loudspeaker. With the spatial separation of the spondees and the noise, the CRISP and CRISP Jr. can also provide an estimate of the spatial release from masking; however, spatial release from masking is not currently a task that is typically assessed preoperatively given the characteristically poor speech recognition performance of pediatric implant candidates.

Speech-Recognition Test Materials in Older Children

Current implant candidacy criteria for older children are based on either mono- or multisyllabic word recognition depending on which is developmentally appropriate for the child being evaluated. The tests that are listed by the cochlear implant manufacturers in their FDA labeling are as follows (presented in order of developmentally appropriate progression): Early Speech Perception (ESP) test (Moog & Geers, 1990), Multisyllabic Lexical Neighborhood Test (MLNT) (Kirk et al., 1995), Lexical Neighborhood Test (LNT) (Kirk et al., 1995), Phonetically Balanced Kindergarten (PBK) word recognition test (Haskins, 1949), and HINT sentences for children (HINT-C) (Gelnett, Sumida, Nilsson, & Soli, 1995).

In addition to the metrics outlined by the manufacturers in the labeled indications, there are a number of other tests available that are appropriate for describing a child's auditory and speech perception profile and may ultimately aid the process of candidate selection. One such metric is the Bamford-Kowal-Bench speech-in-noise test (BKB-SIN; Etymotic Research, Elk Grove Village, Ill; Killion et al., 2001). The BKB-SIN is a sentence recognition task that uses sentences from the BKB corpus (Bench, Kowal, & Bamford, 1979)—the same source used to construct the HINT and HINT-C sentences. The BKB-SIN is a pseudoadaptive metric in that the recorded, multitalker babble automatically increases by 3 dB with each fixed-level sentence in the list. The BKB-SIN provides a raw score, referred to as SNR-50, as well as an estimate of SNR loss. The SNR-50 provides the SNR required for the listener to achieve approximately 50% correct and is based on classic speech perception research describing the determination of SRTs (Tillman & Olsen, 1973). The SNR loss describes the listener's deficit relative to normative data for age-matched subjects with normal hearing. Thus,

the SNR loss provides information about how a child is able to perceive speech in noise relative to his or her peers with normal hearing.

Assessing speech recognition in noise is a reasonable endeavor as children are rarely in quiet listening environments. Current FDA indications, however, do not suggest the use of speech-in-noise testing for determining either adult or pediatric implant candidacy. Educational acoustic research has shown that occupied classroom noise can range from 48 dBA to 69 dBB with the mean level approximately 65 dBA for an early elementary classroom (e.g., Sanders, 1965; Nober & Nober, 1975; Bess, Sinclair, & Riggs, 1984; Finitzo-Hieber, 1988). Considering a child's listening environment both inside and outside the classroom, research has shown that Leq 24-hr measurement averages 87.3 dBA for all students and 95.5 dBA for fifth graders (Clark & Govett, 1995). Given that a child's everyday listening environment is much noisier than even that encountered by the typical adult, it follows that in the process of determining implant candidacy speech recognition in noise should be standard practice. It is likely that a pediatric minimum speech test battery will soon emerge providing pediatric implant audiologists with best-practice recommendations for the minimum testing to be conducted both pre- and post-implant.

Thinking Beyond the "Criteria Checklist" for Pediatric Candidate Selection

Older children assessed with word and sentence recognition testing is required to exhibit considerably lower performance than even that listed for adult FDA implant labeling. Word-recognition candidacy criteria for the older child ranges from 12 to 30% correct in the best-aided condition across the three manufacturers. Advanced Bionics further lists performance up to 30% correct for HINT-C sentences, when developmentally appropriate for children over 4 years. This same manufacturer, however, lists up to 50% HINT sentence recognition performance for adult candidates. One must question the reasoning behind listing disproportionally restrictive criteria for pediatric implant criteria given that children are in the process of acquiring auditory language. It is for this reason that the need for the expansion of pediatric cochlear implant criteria has been and remains to be a hot topic. An ever increasing body of literature has emerged supporting a relatively narrow critical period for cochlear implantation for the development of listening and spoken language (Hayes et al., 2009; Moog & Geers, 2010; Bergeson et al., 2010; Niparko et al., 2010; Habib et al., 2010; Houston & Miyamoto, 2010) as well as auditory pathway maturation (Ponton et al., 2000; Sharma et al., 2002; Eggermont et al., 2003; Gordon et al., 2005; Kral, Tillein, Heid, Klinke, & Hartmann, 2006; Sharma & Dorman, 2006; Gilley, Sharma, & Dorman, 2008; Sharma et al., 2009). It seems reasonable that the combined fields of otology, audiology and speech/language pathology are questioning the reasoning behind labeling the most stringent candidacy criteria for the youngest of auditory language learners and that criterion-level performance should more closely approximate or even exceed that which is outlined for adult implant candidates.

EVALUATION OF AUDITORY SKILLS AND PROGRESS IN INFANTS AND CHILDREN 3 YEARS OF AGE OR LESS

Determining a child's auditory skills and progress with hearing aids prior to determining implant candidacy is not as easy as studying the audiogram. It is well known that similar audiograms do not necessarily yield similar levels of benefit from amplification across a range of hearing losses and configurations. Given that speech-recognition performance cannot be completed for infants and many toddlers, it is critical that the candidacy evaluation process include assessment of auditory skills, development, and progress with hearing aids. From the perspective of the audiologist, these skills will most likely be assessed via parental history and administration of validated questionnaires that are designed to gauge a child's auditory-based responsiveness to sounds in their environment.

One of the most common questionnaires used for children from birth to 3 years is the Infant–Toddler version of the Meaningful Auditory Integration Scale (IT-MAIS) (Zimmerman-Phillips et al., 2000). All three cochlear implant companies make reference to the MAIS (Robbins et al., 1991) and/or IT-MAIS for use in determining auditory progress with amplification. For the youngest of children, the 10-item IT-MAIS is frequently used due to the widespread familiarity of the metric as well as the ease and time required of administration (<10 min). As shown in Figure 3–1, the IT-MAIS is designed to be administered in a structured, parental-interview format and thus requires that the clinician interpret open-ended responses and assign numerical scores ranging from 0 (never) to 4 (always).

Other parental questionnaires designed to assess spontaneous and prompted responsiveness to sound for infants and toddlers have surfaced and are gaining popularity among clinicians. The LittlEars Auditory Questionnaire (MED-EL) (Weichbold et al., 2005; Coninx et al., 2009) is composed of 35 yes/no questions designed to gauge a child's auditory-based responses to different sounds and environments. The questions are organized hierarchically with a progression of difficulty so that the parent can stop answering questions following six consecutive "no" answers.

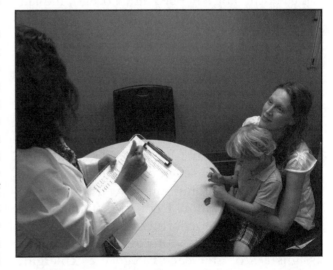

FIGURE 3–1. Shown here is a clinician administering an auditory questionnaire using a parental interview style.

It is designed for use in children up to 24 months of age for normal hearing or 24 months following implantation, though a child with normal development would be expected to reach ceiling levels prior to that test point. Administration of LittlEars takes very little time, and because it does not require parental interview, it does not need to take up time during the actual appointment.

The Auditory Skills Checklist (ASC) (Meinzen-Derr et al., 2007) was developed in response to the increasing number of children being implanted under 12 months of age. The ASC is a 35-item questionnaire that assesses detection, discrimination, identification, and comprehension. Similar to the IT-MAIS, the ASC is designed to be administered in a parental-interview style as well as via clinician observation for which the parent/administrator assigns a rating ranging from 0 to 2 as follows: 0, child does not have the skill; 1, child has demonstrated emerging skill development; and 2, child consistently demonstrates the skill. The ASC can be administered along with the IT-MAIS as it is expected that the ASC can be used over a longer period of time (for children implanted up to 3 years of age) and it provides a detailed multidimensional assessment over smaller increments of auditory-skill development.

Another questionnaire that offers valuable information in the candidacy process, though designed primarily for use following implantation, is the Functioning After Pediatric Cochlear Implantation (FAPCI) questionnaire (Lin et al., 2007). The 23-item FAPCI is considered appropriate for the 2- to 5-year old range and does not require parental interview for administration. Using the FAPCI during the candidacy process provides clinicians and families with a baseline against which future growth in auditory skills can be gauged.

The Functional Auditory Performance Indicators (FAPI) (Stredler-Brown & DeConde Johnson, 2003) assesses seven categories of auditory development including sound awareness, meaningful sounds, auditory feedback, sound localization, discrimination, short-term auditory memory, and linguistic auditory processing. The clinician assigns a score for each category as emerging (0–35%), in process (36–79%), or acquired (80–100%). The FAPI can be used in children as young as a few months of age and can continue to be used until "acquired" scores are obtained for all categories.

The Early Language Milestone scale (ELM) (Coplan, 1987) is a 43-item tool designed to assess language development in children from birth to 3 years. The tool has three sections focusing on expressive, receptive, and visual language. The ELM is typically administered via parental interview and based on parental report; however, there are sections for which clinician observation can also be used. Administration and scoring is estimated in the range of 3–10 min depending on the child's age, level of development, and scoring method (i.e., pass/fail or point scoring).

Individual clinics determine which auditory questionnaires best meet the needs of their patient population and their families. What is more important than the actual questionnaires used is that the clinicians within a given program be consistent across all patients. The cochlear implant team members must closely monitor the auditory progress of children during the hearing aid trial period, being careful to describe and analyze a child's complete auditory profile and not fall into the trap of failing to see "beyond the audiogram."

EVALUATION OF AUDITORY SKILLS AND PROGRESS IN PRESCHOOL TO SCHOOL-AGE CHILDREN

As with infants and toddlers, assessment of auditory skills and development for older children may not be well predicted by the audiogram. Although behavioral assessment of auditory skills should always be attempted for preschool- and school-age children, due to a number of factors, behavioral assessment may not be possible or only very limited information may be obtained. For this reason, there are several auditory-skill questionnaires designed for use with preschool and school-age children.

The Meaningful Auditory Integration Scale (MAIS) (Robbins et al., 1991) is a 10-item parental-interview-style questionnaire designed for assessing auditory skills including spontaneous responses to sounds for children age 3–5 years. All three cochlear implant manufacturers make reference to this questionnaire for determining auditory progress—or lack thereof—with appropriately fitted amplification.

The Parents' Evaluation of Aural/Oral Performance of Children (PEACH) is a 13-item questionnaire designed for parental estimation of the child's functional aural and oral abilities in everyday life (Ching & Hill, 2007). It is considered appropriate for children age 3–7 years. The PEACH requires parents to reflect on their child's listening behavior over the previous week and assigns a numerical value to parental answers ranging from 0 (never or 0%) to 4 (always or 75–100%). The PEACH includes questions relating to listening in both quiet and noisy surroundings.

The 23-item FAPCI questionnaire (Lin et al., 2007) can be administered to parents of children age 2–5 years. As stated previously, although the FAPCI was originally intended to track postoperative progress, using it during the candidacy process provides clinicians and families with a baseline against which future growth in auditory skills can be gauged.

There are other general parent-based questionnaires available for use with children who have severe-to-profound sensory hearing loss including Meaningful Use of Speech Sounds (MUSS) (Robbins et al., 1998), Children's Home Inventory for Listening Difficulties (CHILD) (Anderson & Smaldino, 1999), and Developmental Index of Audition and Listening (DIAL) (Palmer & Mormer, 1999). The questionnaires listed in Table 3–2 are those most frequently used with children both pre- and post-implantation. More important than the actual questionnaires used, however, is that individual clinics determine the appropriateness of the different instruments for their patient population. What is most important is consistency across clinicians and patients within a cochlear implant program so that individual clinics can track the typical performance for children implanted at their center.

Testing Conditions

As mentioned in Chapter 2, the testing conditions for determining cochlear implant candidacy are not widely agreed upon among clinicians. All implant manufacturers reference the "best-aided condition" for determining adult and pediatric candidacy. Clinicians may interpret the term "best-aided condition" differently. In the case of asymmetric hearing loss and/or speech recognition performance across the ears, the best-aided condition may be a gross overestimation of performance as compared with performance for the proposed ear to be implanted. Fabry et al. (2009) recommended individual ear testing for postoperative assessment of performance with adult candidates; thus, it follows that if we are to more closely approximate adult candidacy for children learning language, we should also be assessing individual ear performance for pediatric implant candidates. It is important to note, however, that it may not be possible to obtain individual ear estimates of speech recognition, particularly not in the same assessment visit. Nevertheless, it should remain a goal and one that is critical for children with asymmetric hearing loss.

Hearing Aids: Trial, Verification, and Evaluation of Speech and Language

The speech/language pathologist (SLP) plays a critical role in the cochlear implant candidate selection process for infants and children. Often a child presenting for cochlear implant evaluation has little or no language in terms of either manual or spoken communication abilities. The evaluation of speech, and perhaps more importantly language, should be scheduled to coincide with a prior audiology appointment so that the hearing aid settings are verified. According to the American Academy of Audiology's Pediatric Amplification Protocol (2003), best practices requires that hearing aids be verified using either probe-microphone measurements or test-box verification with patient-specific real ear to coupler difference (RECD) corrections. Furthermore, given that nonlinear hearing aid circuitry is generally used to attain audibility at various input levels, a prescriptive formula, such as DSL m[i/o] (Seewald et al., 1985; Cornelisse, Seewald, & Jamieson, 1995; Scollie et al., 2005), should be used to verify target audibility at speech-input levels corresponding to soft, average, and loud, such as 50, 60, and 70 dB SPL.

Table 3–2. Questionnaires Most Frequently Used with Children Both Pre- and Post-Implantation

Measure Name	Length and Estimated Time to Complete	Domains Assessed	Age Range	Administration
LittlEARS[a]	35 yes/no items; 5–7 min	Age appropriateness of auditory behaviors (e.g., responsiveness to acoustic rituals, looking for sound sources)	0–24 months	Independent parental completion; parental report
Auditory Skills Checklist	35 items; <10 min	Detection, discrimination, identification, and comprehension	0–36 months	Parental interview; clinician observation
Early Language Milestones (ELM)	43 items; <10 min	Auditory-based language behaviors (expressive, receptive, and visual)	0–36 months	Parental report; direct observation
Infant–Toddler Meaningful Auditory Integration Scale (IT-MAIS)	10 items; 5–10 min	Device bonding, alerting to sound, vocalization, deriving meaning from sound	0–36 months	Parental interview
Functioning After Pediatric Cochlear Implantation (FAPCI)	23 items; 5–10 min	Speech intelligibility, auditory responsiveness, real-world verbal communication	2–5 years	Independent parental completion; parental report
Functional Auditory Performance Indicators (FAPI)	33 items; 10–15 min	Auditory awareness, feedback and integration, discrimination, comprehension, memory, and linguistic processing	3 months until "acquired" is obtained for all categories	Parental interview; parental report; direct observation
Meaningful Auditory Integration Scale (MAIS)	10 items; 5–10 min	Device bonding, alerting to sound, vocalization, deriving meaning from sound	3–5 years	Parental interview
Parents' Evaluation of Aural/Oral Performance of Children (PEACH)	13 items; 5–10 min	Aural/oral speech communicative behaviors in quiet and noisy situations	3–7 years	Independent parental completion; parental report

[a]MED-EL, Barnsley, UK

When beginning a hearing aid trial for infants who are thought to meet cochlear implant candidacy based on the severity of the hearing loss, it is critical to also schedule a speech/language assessment to determine baseline language skills against which future development can be measured. The specific metrics used by the SLP are dependent on both the chronologic age as well as the "hearing" age of the child (see Chapter 4). During the hearing aid trial period, it is expected that the child make *at least* month-for-month progress in auditory skills as well as speech and language developmental progress with amplification in order to derive appropriate benefit from hearing aids. What that means is that if a child has been fitted with hearing aids for 6 months, they should make *at least* 6 months of progress in auditory skills and speech/language development. If this is not the case for a child making full-time use of amplification and appropriate intervention—in the absence of developmental delay and/or cognitive concerns—then cochlear implantation must be considered.

It is expected that a child receive at least two speech/language evaluations during the candidacy selection process during the hearing aid trial. Although it may not be possible to administer norm-referenced measures over such a short period of time (see Chapter 8), there are many criterion-referenced measures that are available and can provide valuable information about a child's progress with appropriately fitted hearing aids.

It is crucial that children receive appropriate intervention including regular visits from a member of the early intervention team, speech/language therapy, as well as active parental involvement to supplement therapy with proper modeling of spoken-language development. The cochlear implant team can glean considerable information from parental compliance to not only full-time use of amplification, but also to the recommended therapy schedule during the candidacy selection process. It sets an important precedent for what will be expected following cochlear implant surgery, as intensive intervention and therapy will be required if the child is to make full use of the audibility provided by the new, electrical signal. More detailed information regarding the role of the SLP in the determination of pediatric cochlear implant candidacy is provided in Chapter 4.

Role of the Social Worker and/or Psychologist in the Determination of Cochlear Implant Candidacy

The role of the social worker and/or psychologist in the determination of cochlear implant candidacy can be extremely valuable for pediatric candidates and their families. A psychological evaluation, particularly a developmental psychological evaluation, may be recommended by the cochlear implant team in the event that concerns are raised regarding the overall cognitive and global developmental functioning of the child. Other areas in which a psychologist and/or social worker can provide valuable assistance is for families struggling with the diagnosis and implications of having a child who will be dependent on technology for hearing and communication. Other areas within the scope of the psychologist and/or social worker in determining implant candidacy include evaluation of family dynamics and level of dedication to the recommended postoperative therapy schedule. Such guidance can be sought after and/or recommended by the cochlear implant team pre- and post-implant, as needed.

An additional area in which a social worker can provide counseling and support for families is that of finances as related to medical care surrounding aural habilitation. Families may be unaware of the financial resources available to them for insurance coverage of medical care, therapy, and assistive listening devices. Social workers not only provide this information but also help provide access to the appropriate paperwork and help families navigate through the application processes, which can be daunting. In some cases, social workers can help families coordinate medical and therapy appointments as well as review the past and current schedule of appointments to ensure that all medical specialties and evaluations have been made available to the family.

MEDICAL AND SURGICAL ISSUES

The cochlear implant surgeon, typically an otologist or neuro-otologist, clearly plays a vital role in the determination of implant candidacy. Surgeons perform a thorough preoperative examination in addition to being responsible for the surgical procedure and postoperative otologic medical care. The otologist and his or her medical team also ensure that all cochlear implant candidates are current on recommended immunizations prior to surgery. The recommended immunization schedule for children undergoing cochlear implantation can be found on the Centers for Disease Control website (http://www.cdc.gov/vaccines/vpd-vac/mening/cochlear/dis-cochlear-gen.htm) and includes, at a minimum, an age-specific pneumococcal vaccination. For children up to 18 years of age, the pneumococcal conjugate vaccination is marketed under the name Prevnar 13 (Wyeth Pharmaceuticals [Pfizer], New York, N.Y.), and at the time of chapter preparation, it protects against 13 strains of pneumococcal infection. For children over 5–6 years of age, physicians may also recommend pneumococcal conjugate vaccine 23 (PCV23 or Pneumovax 23, Merck & Co., West Point, PA), which is known to protect against 23 of the most common strains of pneumococcal infection.

As with adult candidates, the otologist orders a preanesthetic medical evaluation or preoperative evaluation to ensure that the candidate is able to undergo surgery and the associated anesthetic risk. The preoperative evaluation includes assessment of vital signs and general medical evaluation to identify the presence of health problems which may affect peri- and/or postanesthetic care. Furthermore, the otologist typically refers children to ophthalmology as well as medical genetics, because approximately 40% of children with sensorineural hearing loss have other medical and/or developmental comorbidities including cognitive, visual, motor, behavioral, and learning (Fortnum et al., 2002; Gallaudet Research Institute, 2008; Roberts & Hindley, 1999; Van Naarden et al., 1999). The otologist also refers to additional medical specialties such as neurology, physical medicine and rehabilitation, and developmental pediatrics, as needed.

Otologists also routinely order imaging studies including computed tomography (CT) and/or magnetic resonance imaging (MRI) to determine cochlear patency as well as to rule out cochlear or other temporal bone anomalies that could impact the surgical insertion of the device. Cochlear and temporal bone anomalies are not necessarily contraindicated for cochlear implantation; however, preoperative awareness of such issues provides the best preparation for implant device selection and proposed surgical technique. High-resolution CT is generally ordered for all patients having met audiologic criteria for cochlear implantation. MRI is generally ordered for pediatric patients who have exhibited no behavioral hearing via audiometric testing and/or who are suspect for cochlear nerve deficiency. It is within the protocol for many cochlear implant programs that MRI is ordered for all pediatric patients prior to implantation. Given that postoperative MRI above 0.3 T is currently contraindicated in the United States *without* magnet removal (see physician package inserts), many otologists consider preoperative MRI valuable as a last chance to obtain detailed imaging information regarding the cochleovestibular nerve.

UTILITY OF PREDICTIVE VARIABLES FOR POSTOPERATIVE OUTCOMES

Once a family is informed that their child is a candidate for cochlear implantation, in-depth counseling and education is critical. Just as discussed in Chapter 2 for adult candidates, pre-implant counseling is directly within the scope of the audiologist and constitutes a significant portion of each pediatric cochlear implant evaluation. As important as educating the family about the function of cochlear implants and what they do is the focus on what implants *cannot* do, such as restore "normal" hearing and auditory function.

Perhaps the most frequent question that families ask regarding cochlear implantation for their child is how well he or she will do with listening and spoken language—particularly with respect to a child's normal-hearing peers. There are a number of potential factors affecting postoperative outcomes, including wear time, intervention, pre-implant audiometric thresholds, integrity of cochlear and neural structures, and etiology.

Age at Implantation

Age at implantation directly affects outcomes. As mentioned previously, there is a growing body of literature documenting a relatively narrow critical period for cochlear implantation for the development of listening and spoken language

(Hayes et al., 2009; Moog & Geers, 2010; Bergeson et al., 2010; Niparko et al., 2010; Habib et al., 2010; Houston & Miyamoto, 2010) as well as auditory pathway maturation (Ponton et al., 2000; Sharma et al., 2002; Eggermont et al., 2003; Gordon et al., 2005; Kral et al., 2006; Sharma & Dorman, 2006; Gilley et al., 2008; Sharma et al., 2009). Houston and colleagues have shown significantly better word learning abilities in infants implanted under 13 months of age (Houston et al., 2012; Houston & Miyamoto, 2010) as compared to children implanted between 16 and 23 months of age. Other studies have shown that children implanted in the range of 18–24 months of age demonstrate significantly greater language and vocabulary development—both expressive and receptive—than children implanted over 2 years of age (Hayes et al., 2009; Niparko et al., 2010; Artières, Vieu, Mondain, Uziel & Venail, 2011; Markman, Quittner, Eisenberg, Tobey, Thal, & Niparko, 2011; Boons et al., 2012).

Despite the relationship between age at implantation and auditory/oral language outcomes, children implanted over 18–24 months of age still derive significant benefit; however, family counseling regarding expectations needs to be realistic with the child's age at activation noted as a critical variable. In other words, clinicians should counsel that more aggressive intervention might be needed for the child implanted over 2 years of age for whom the family's goal remains auditory/oral language with high levels of speech intelligibility.

Wear Time

Cochlear implants provide access to sound for children; however, the processor(s) must be worn all waking hours in order to derive maximum benefit. The Alexander Graham Bell Association for the Deaf and Hard of Hearing has provided powerful examples highlighting the need for consistent device use. An infant with normal hearing typically listens for 10 hr per day totaling at least 3,650 hr of listening over the first year of life. For the infant making only part-time use of hearing aids during the candidacy process (estimated at 4 hr per day) it would take 6 years to provide as much listening experience as that of a baby with normal hearing or a baby who wears hearing aids and/or implant sound processors all waking hours (Stovall, 1982; Rossi, 2003). A toddler/preschooler with normal hearing is estimated to be listening approximately 12 hr per day. Over the course of a year, that equals 4,380 hr of listening. For the toddler/preschooler wearing the implant sound processors on a part-time basis, such as 2.75 hr per day while at preschool, it would take 9 years to provide as much listening experience that is gained over a single year for the child with normal hearing or the child making full-time use of the sound processors (Rossi, 2003).

Although age at implantation is a critical variable regarding outcomes, if full-time usage of the sound processor(s) is not enforced, *progress will not be made*. The importance of wear time is a critical counseling tool and one that stands repeating multiple times during preoperative counseling as well as at postoperative follow-up appointments.

Intervention

The best outcomes are not simply achieved with early implantation and processor wear time. It has been repeatedly documented that the highest levels of auditory/oral language outcomes are achieved in conjunction with early and consistent intervention (e.g., Nicholas & Geers, 2007; Geers, Moog, Biedenstein, Brenner, & Hayes 2009; Moeller, 2000; Moog & Geers, 2010). Higher levels of receptive and expressive language of school-age children with cochlear implants are associated with early enrollment in comprehensive intervention programs including those incorporating parental/family involvement and focusing on listening and spoken language (Moeller, 2000; Moog & Geers, 2010). It must be stressed to families that the work does not end with the surgical placement of the implant. In other words, cochlear implants do not "cure" hearing loss. Rather, the hardest work begins once the implant has been activated. The best outcomes are achieved with intensive habilitation including regular speech/language therapy, continuation of infant and family services with home-based infant/family specialists, enrollment in parent–infant programs, and later involvement in a preschool program focusing on listening and spoken language; thus, it is actually the case that implant surgery and activation represent only the first steps in the journey.

It is noteworthy that an auditory/oral approach to communication may not be the goal of every family, nor may it be a reasonable expectation based on the age of identification, age at implantation, family dynamics, and/or other developmental delays associated with the underlying etiology or comorbidities. There are other modes of communication incorporating signing, cued speech, augmentative communication, or any combination thereof. Keeping the family's goals in view is paramount, with an eye toward reasonable expectations, which will allow for the highest level of family-centered counseling and overall satisfaction.

Preimplant Audiometric Thresholds

Audiologists and surgeons tend to place considerable emphasis on the audiogram and audiometric thresholds; however, while the audiogram represents a diagnostic measure of an individual's auditory detection or *sensation*, it does not always accurately reflect an individual's auditory function or *perception*—particularly not for children with congenital hearing loss. Given that children receiving cochlear implants typically have bilateral severe-to-profound hearing loss, there exists a very narrow range of preoperative audiometric thresholds with which to correlate postoperative performance. As discussed in Chapter 2, for adult predictive variables of postoperative performance, there are no studies which show a relationship between preoperative audiometric thresholds and postoperative outcomes for pediatric implant recipients.

Integrity of Cochlear and Neural Structures

Any structural anomaly involving the bony labyrinth, cochlear lumen, or internal auditory canal has the potential to affect postoperative outcomes. It has been stated that up to 35% of children with sensorineural hearing loss have cochleovestibular anomalies (Papsin, 2005). Common structural abnormalities that one might expect to uncover in the pediatric population include Mondini dysplasia, common cavity, enlarged vestibular aqueduct, and atretic internal auditory canal. All of these diagnoses are observable via CT and would thus be diagnosed prior to implantation for pediatric candidates, provided that the temporal bone CT protocol had been completed.

Cochlear nerve deficiency (CND) is another structural abnormality that may be discovered for a child diagnosed with profound sensorineural hearing loss. CND refers to cases in which the auditory nerve is either absent or hypoplastic. In cases of CND for which the auditory nerve is absent, cochlear implantation is contraindicated because the presence of an auditory nerve is a vital prerequisite given that the primary auditory neurons, located within the modiolus and generally referred to as spiral ganglion cells, are the targets for electrical stimulation via the implanted intracochlear electrodes. Cases of CND for which the auditory nerve is hypoplastic are associated with poorer postoperative outcomes; however, cochlear implantation can offer significant communicative benefit not realized via amplification (Teagle et al., 2010; Buchman et al., 2011; Seymour et al., 2010). CND is observable via MRI and would be diagnosed prior to implantation for pediatric candidates, provided that MRI with the temporal bone protocol had been completed.

Auditory neuropathy is another issue that may affect postoperative outcomes. Auditory neuropathy can manifest as a true neuropathy of cranial nerve VIII, which is generally observed along with other peripheral neuropathies, or an auditory neuropathy spectrum disorder (ANSD)—the latter of which is frequently associated with pediatric cases of auditory neuropathy. For more details on the audiometric profile characteristic of ANSD, see Chapter 2.

Auditory neuropathy including peripheral nerve damage has the potential to negatively impact outcomes; in fact, peripheral auditory neuropathy would preclude cochlear implant candidacy as the criterion of intact auditory nerve would not be met. However, it is often difficult to definitively diagnose auditory neuropathy from ANSD preoperatively—particularly for very young children—and thus our counseling and expectations need to recognize the possibility. True auditory nerve is quite rare in the pediatric population such that when present, it is most frequently a diagnosis secondary to a primary peripheral neuropathy such as that associated with Charcot-Marie-Tooth disease.

Etiology

Just as with adult patients, the etiology of hearing loss for a large proportion of pediatric patients is largely unknown. It is estimated that approximately half of all congenital hearing losses have an underlying genetic component, though this estimate will likely increase as human genome research continues (Rehm, 2005). For a large proportion of pediatric patients, there is generally no concern about etiology affecting counseling for postoperative outcomes. There are, however, some etiologies which are known to potentially affect postoperative outcomes for pediatric cochlear implant recipients. Although certainly not exhaustive, the most common etiologies and associated concerns regarding outcomes are covered here.

Meningitis

The incidence of bacterial meningitis is significantly higher in children than in adults and accounts for approximately 6% of cases of acquired sensorineural hearing loss in childhood (Smith et al., 2005). The pneumococcal conjugate vaccine has significantly reduced the incidence of bacterial meningitis in children; however, for those that do contract meningitis, approximately 5–10% of cases experience severe-to-profound sensorineural hearing loss (Baraff, Lee, & Schriger, 1993; Smith et al., 2005). As mentioned in Chapter 2, the underlying cause of hearing loss associated with bacterial meningitis is the development of labyrinthitis, loss of hair cells, spiral ganglion cell degeneration, and cochlear ossification (Lu & Schuknecht, 1994; Nadol & Hsu, 1991). See Chapter 2 for more information regarding meningitis and projected outcomes.

Syndrome-Related Deafness

There are a number of syndromes known to be associated with various degrees of sensorineural hearing loss. There are numerous reports of successful outcomes with cochlear implantation in children with syndromic hearing loss including branchial-oto-renal syndrome, CHARGE syndrome, Pendred syndrome, Refsum disease, Usher syndrome, and Waardeburg syndrome (e.g., Loundon, Marlin, Busquet, Denoyelle, Roger, Renaud, & Garabedian 2003; Raine, Kurukulasuriva, Bajaj, & Strachan, 2008; Cullen, Zdanski, Roush, Brown, Teagle, Pillsbury, & Buchman, C. 2006; Vescan, Parnes, Cucci, Smith, & MacNeill, 2002; Arndt et al., 2010; Lina-Granade, Porot, Vesson, & Truy, 2010). Those syndromes known also to be related to progressive loss of vision, such as Usher syndrome and Refsum disease, can particularly affect outcomes as speech/language therapy makes use of visual cues. Even auditory/oral language development has a strong nonverbal component, and thus early implantation prior to the onset of significant visual loss is recommended. Syndromes having the potential to impact global development and cognition, such as CHARGE, also expectedly impact outcomes and thus require extensive preimplant counseling regarding appropriate expectations.

Chromosome-Related Deafness

The chromosomal condition most commonly linked with sensorineural hearing loss is Trisomy 21, more commonly referred to as Down syndrome. Down syndrome is associated with sensorineural hearing loss in approximately 5–20% of cases with severe-to-profound deafness present in 5% or fewer cases (Roizen, Wolters, Nicol, & Blondis, 1993; Hans, England, Prowse, Young, & Sheehan, 2010). For those children with Down syndrome and significant sensorineural hearing loss, however, cochlear implantation remains a viable treatment option (Hans et al., 2010). Expectations for progress following cochlear implantation are directly related to the cognitive status of the individual, which can vary widely with Down syndrome, as well as the increased risk for middle ear disease. Given the propensity for middle ear disease in children with Down syndrome, it is particularly important that appropriate vaccinations are up to date.

Other Variables Affecting Postoperative Outcomes

In recent years there have been several multicenter longitudinal studies examining postoperative outcomes for pediatric implant recipients (e.g., Niparko et al., 2010; Barker et al., 2009; Geers, Brenner, & Davidson, 2003; Szagun & Stumper, 2012). Other than the expected variables, such as duration of hearing loss prior to implantation, age at implantation, early intervention, educational placement, postoperative degree of audibility with implants, and others, there are a number of associated variables related to family/social issues. Those variables found to be related to outcomes for language development and speech recognition are family size, intelligence, socioeconomic status, maternal level of education, and the amount of time spent talking to the child at home (sometimes referred to as language exposure). Some of these predictive variables, such as family size, maternal level of education, and socioeconomic status, are not necessarily appropriate to discuss during preoperative counseling. The variable that should be discussed at length by the audiologist, speech/language pathologist, deaf educator, and early-intervention specialist is the amount of time spent talking to the child at home. These behaviors should be started well before the surgery date, setting a precedent and learned behavior/habit of incorporating language modeling and functional auditory/oral communication throughout the day.

CONCLUSION

Cochlear implants have been shown to literally change the course of a child's life potentially allowing for normal development of speech, language, and literacy. Even for those children not able to achieve an auditory/oral approach to speech and language, cochlear implants provide sound awareness increasing safety and quality of life for the recipient. It is important to recognize that pediatric candidacy criteria have dramatically evolved over the past several decades, and that cochlear implants are no longer only for children with profound deafness. The interdisciplinary cochlear implant team offers patients the highest level of care and information needed to progress through the candidacy selection process.

REFERENCES

American Academy of Audiology. (2003). *Pediatric amplification protocol*. Retrieved May 2, 2012, from http://www.audiology.org

Anderson, K., & Smaldino, J. (1999). Listening inventories for education: A classroom measurement tool. *The Hearing Journal, 52*(10), 74–75.

Arndt, A., Laszig, R., Beck, R., Schild, C., Maier, W., Birkenhager, R., et al. (2010). Spectrum of hearing disorders and their management in children with CHARGE syndrome. *Otology & Neurotology, 31*, 67–73.

Artières, F., Vieu, A., Mondain, M., Uziel, A., & Venail, F. (2009). Impact of early cochlear implantation on the linguistic development of the deaf child. *Otology & Neurotology, 30*(6), 736–742.

Baraff, L. J., Lee, S. I., & Schriger, D. L. (1993). Outcomes of bacterial meningitis in children: a meta-analysis. *Pediatric Infections and Disorders Journal, 12*(5), 389–394.

Barker, D. H., Quittner, A. L., Fink, N. E., Eisenberg, L. S., Tobey, E. A., & Niparko, J. K. (2009). CDaCI Investigative Team. Predicting behavior problems in deaf and hearing children: The influences of language, attention, and parent-child communication. *Developmental Psychopathology, 21*(2), 373–392.

Bench, J., Kowal, A., & Bamford, J. (1979). The BKB (Bamford-Kowal-Bench) sentence lists for partially-hearing children. *British Journal of Audiology, 13*(3), 108–112.

Bergeson, T. R., Houston, D. M., & Miyamoto, R. T. (2010). Effects of congenital hearing loss and cochlear implantation on audiovisual speech perception in infants and children. *Restorative Neurology and Neuroscience, 28*, 157–165.

Bess, F. H., Sinclair, J. S, & Riggs, D. (1984) Group amplification in schools for the hearing impaired. *Ear and Hearing, 5*, 138–144.

Buchman, C. A., Teagle, H. R., Roush, P. A., Park, L. R., Hatch, D., Woodard, J., et al. (2011). Cochlear implantation in children with labyrinthine anomalies and cochlear nerve deficiency: Implications for auditory brainstem implantation. *Laryngoscope, 121,* 1979–1988.

Boons, T., Brokx, J. P., Dhooge, I., Frijns, J. H., Peeraer, L., Vermeulen, A., et al. (2012). Predictors of spoken language development following pediatric cochlear implantation. *Ear and Hearing,* May 2 [Epub ahead of print].

Carhart, R. (1946). Monitored live-voice as a test of auditory acuity. *Journal of the Acoustical Society of America, 17,* 339–349.

Ching, T. Y., & Hill, M. (2007). The parents' evaluation of aural/oral performance of children (PEACH) scale: Normative data. *Journal of the American Academy of Audiology, 18*(3), 220–235.

Clark, W.W, & Govett, S. B. (1995). *School-related noise exposure in children.* Paper presented at the Association for Research in Otolaryngology Mid-Winter Meeting, St. Petersburg, FL.

Coninx, F., Weichbold, V., Tsiakpini, L., Autrique, E., Bescond, G., Tamas, L., et al. (2009). Validation of the LittlEARS auditory questionnaire in children with normal hearing. *International Journal of Pediatric Otorhinolaryngology, 73*(12), 1761–1768.

Coplan, J. (1987). *ELM scale: The early language milestone scale.* Austin, TX: Pro-Ed.

Cornelisse, L., Seewald, R., & Jamieson, D. (1995). The input/output formula: a theoretical approach to the fitting of personal amplification devices. *Journal of the Acoustical Society of America, 97*(3), 1854–1864.

Cullen, R. D., Zdanski, C., Roush P, Brown, C., Teagle, H., Pillsbury, H., & Buchman, C. (2006). Cochlear implants in Waardenburg syndrome. *Laryngoscope, 116,* 1273–1275.

Elliott, L. L., & Katz, D. (1980). *Development of a new children's test of speech discrimination* (Technical manual). St. Louis, MO: Auditec.

Finitzo-Hieber, T. (1988). Classroom acoustics. In R. Roeser (Ed.), *Auditory disorders in school children* (2nd ed., pp. 221–223). New York, NY: Thieme-Stratton.

Gallaudet Research Institute. (2008). *Regional and national summary report of data from the 2008 annual survey of deaf and hard of hearing children and youth.* Washington, DC: Gallaudet University.

Gelnett, D., Sumida, A., Nilsson, M., & Soli, S. D. (1995). *Development of the Hearing-in-Noise Test for Children (HINT-C).* Paper presented at the annual meeting of the American Academy of Audiology, Dallas, TX.

Geers, A., Brenner, C., & Davidson, L. (2003). Factors associated with development of speech perception skills in children implanted by age five. *Ear and Hearing, 24,* 24S–35S.

Geers, A. E., Moog, J. S., Biedenstein, J., Brenner, C., & Hayes, H. (2009). Spoken language scores of children using cochlear implants compared to hearing age-mates at school entry. *Journal of Deaf Studies and Deaf Education, 14,* 371–385.

Gilley, P. M., Sharma, A., & Dorman, M. F. (2008). Cortical reorganization in children with cochlear implants. *Brain Research, 1239,* 56–65.

Gravel, J. S., White, K. R., Johnson, J. L., Widen, J. E., Vohr, B. R., James, M., et al. (2005). A multisite study to examine the efficacy of the otoacoustic emission/automated auditory brainstem response newborn hearing screening protocol: Recommendations for policy, practice, and research. *American Journal of Audiology, 14*(2), S217–S228.

Habib, M. G. , Waltzman, S. B., Tajudeen, B., & Svirsky, M. A. (2010). Speech production intelligibility of early implanted pediatric cochlear implant users. *International Journal of Pediatric Otorhinolaryngology, 74,* 855–859

Hans, P. S., England, R., Prowse, S., Young, E., & Sheehan, P. Z. (2010). UK and Ireland experience of cochlear implants in children with Down syndrome. *International Journal of Pediatric Otorhinolaryngology, 74,* 260–264.

Haskins, H. (1949). *A phonetically balanced test of speech discrimination for children.* Unpublished master's thesis. Northwestern University, Evanston, IL.

Hayes, H., Geers, A. E., Treiman, R., & Moog, J. S. (2009). Receptive vocabulary development in deaf children with cochlear implants: achievement in an intensive auditory-oral educational setting. *Ear and Hearing, 30,* 128–135.

Houston, D. M., & Jusczyk, P. W. (2003). Infants' long-term memory for the sound patterns of words and voices. *Journal of Experimental Psychology: Human Perception and Performance, 29*(6), 1143–1154.

Houston, D. M., & Miyamoto, R. T. (2010). Effects of early auditory experience on word learning and speech perception in deaf children with cochlear implants: Implications for sensitive periods of language development. *Otology & Neurotology, 31,* 1248–1253.

Houston, D. M., Stewart, J., Moberly, A., Hollich, G., & Miyamoto, R. T., (2012). Word learning in deaf children with cochlear implants: Effects of early auditory experience. *Developmental Science, 15,* 448–461.

Jusczyk, P. W., & Hohne, E. A. (1997). Infants' memory for spoken words. *Science, 277*(5334), 1984–1986.

Killion, M., Niquette, P., Revit, L., & Skinner, M. (2001). Quick SIN and BKB-SIN, two new speech-in-noise tests permitting SNR-50 estimates in 1 to 2 min (A). *Journal of the Acoustical Society of America, 109*(5), 2502–2502.

Kim, L. S., Jeong, S. W., Lee, Y. M., & Kim, J. S. (2010). Cochlear implantation in children. *Auris Nasus Larynx, 37*(1), 6–17.

Kirk, K. I., Pisoni, D. B., & Osberger, M. J. (1995). Lexical effects on spoken word recognition by pediatric cochlear implant users. *Ear and Hearing, 16,* 470–481.

Kral, A., Tillein, J., Heid, S., Klinke, R., & Hartmann R. (2006). Cochlear implants: Cortical plasticity in congenital deprivation. *Progress in Brain Research, 157,* 283–313.

Kruel, E., Bell, D., & Nixon, J. (1969). Factors affecting speech discrimination test difficulty. *Journal of Speech and Hearing Research, 12,* 281–287.

Lin, F. R., Ceh, K., Bervinchak, D., Riley, A., Miech, R., & Niparko, J. K. (2007). Development of a communicative performance scale for pediatric cochlear implantation. *Ear and Hearing, 28*(5), 703–712.

Lina-Granade, G., Porot, M., Vesson, J. F., & Truy, E. (2010). More about cochlear implantation in children with CHARGE association. *Cochlear Implants International, 11*(Suppl 1), 187–191.

Loundon, N., Marlin, S., Busquet, D., Denoyelle, F., Roger, G., Renaud, F., & Garabedian, E. N. (2003). Usher syndrome and cochlear implantation. *Otology & Neurotology, 24,* 216–221.

Lu, C. B., & Schuknecht, H. F. (1994). Pathology of prelingual profound deafness: Magnitude of labyrinthitis fibro-ossificans. *American Journal of Otology, 15,* 74–85.

Markman, T. M., Quittner, A. L., Eisenberg, L. S., Tobey, E. A., Thal, D., Niparko, J. K., et al. The CDaCI Investigative Team. (2011). Language development after cochlear implantation: an epigenetic model. *Journal of Neurodevelopmental Disorders, 3*(4), 388–404.

Moeller, M. P. (2000). Early intervention and language development in children who are deaf and hard of hearing. *Pediatrics, 106,* E43.

Moog, J. S., & Geers, A. (1990). *Early speech perception test for profoundly hearing-impaired children.* St. Louis, MO: Central Institute for the Deaf.

Moog, J. S., & Geers, A. E. (2010). Early educational placement and later language outcomes for children with cochlear implants. *Otology & Neurotology, 31,* 1315–1319.

Nadol, J. B. Jr., & Hsu, W. C. (1991). Histopathologic correlation of spiral ganglion cell count and new bone formation in the cochlea following meningogenic labyrinthitis and deafness. *Annals of Otology, Rhinology and Laryngology, 100*(9 Pt 1), 712–716.

Nichani, J., Green, K., Hans, P., Bruce, I., Henderson, L., & Ramsden, R. (2011). Cochlear implantation after bacterial meningitis in children: Outcomes in ossified and nonossified cochleas. *Otology & Neurotology, 32*(5), 784–789.

Nicholas, J. G. & Geers, A. E. (2007). Will they catch up? The role of age at cochlear implantation in the spoken language development of children with severe to profound hearing loss. *Journal of Speech Language Hearing Research, 50*(4), 1048–1062.

Nilsson, M. J., & McCaw, V. M., & Soli S. (1996). *Minimum speech test battery for adult cochlear implant users* (User manual). Los Angeles, CA: House Ear Institute.

Nilsson, M., Soli, S., & Sullivan J. (1994). Development of the Hearing in Noise Test for the measurement of speech reception thresholds in quiet and in noise. *Journal of the Acoustical Society of America, 95,* 1085–1099.

Nober, L. W., & Nober, E. H. (1975) Auditory discrimination of learning disabled children in quiet and classroom noise. *Journal of Learning Disabilities, 8,* 656–659.

Novak, M. A., Black, J. M., & Koch, D. B. (2007). Standard cochlear implantation of adults with residual low-frequency hearing: Implications for combined electro-acoustic stimulation. *Otology & Neurotology, 28*(5), 609–614.

Olsen, W. O. (1998). Average speech levels and spectra in various speaking/listening conditions: A summary of the Pearson, Bennett & Fidel Report (1977). *American Journal of Audiology, 7,* 21–25.

Palmer, C. V., & Mormer, E. (1999) Goals and expectations of the hearing aid fitting. *Trends in Amplification, 4*(2), 61–71.

Papsin, B. C., & Gordon, K. A. (2008). Bilateral cochlear implants should be the standard for children with bilateral sensorineural deafness. *Current Opinion in Otolaryngology & Head and Neck Surgery, 16,* 69–74.

Patrick, D. L., & Erickson, P. (1993). *Health status and health policy: Quality of life in health care evaluation and resource allocation.* New York, NY: Oxford University Press.

Pearsons, K. S., Bennett, R. L., & Fidell, S. (1977). *Speech levels in various noise environments* (Report No. EPA-600/1-77-025). Washington, DC: U.S. Environmental Protection Agency.

Peterson, G. E., & Lehiste, I. (1962). Revised CNC lists for auditory tests. *Journal of Speech and Hearing Disorders, 27,* 62–72.

Peterson, A., Shallop, J., Driscoll, C., Breneman, A., Babb, J., Stoeckel, R., et al. (2003). Outcomes of cochlear implantation in children with auditory neuropathy. *Journal of the American Academy of Audiology, 14*, 188–201.

Ponton, C. W., Eggermont, J. J., Don, M., Waring, M. D., Kwong, B., Cunningham, J., et al. (2000). Maturation of the mismatch negativity: Effects of profound deafness and cochlear implant use. *Audiology and Neurotology, 5*(3–4), 167–185.

Raine, C. H., Kurukulasuriva, M. F., Bajaj, Y., & Strachan, D. R. (2008). Cochlear implantation in Refsum's disease. *Cochlear Implants International, 9*, 97–102.

Rance, G., & Barker, E. J. (2008). Speech perception in children with auditory neuropathy/dyssynchrony managed with either hearing aids or cochlear implants. *Otology & Neurotology, 29*, 179–182.

Rance, G., Beer, D. E., Cone-Wesson, B., Shepherd, R. K., Dowell, R. C., King, A. M., et al. (1999). Clinical findings for a group of infants and young children with auditory neuropathy. *Ear and Hearing, 20*, 238–252.

Rehm, H. L. (2005). A genetic approach to the child with sensorineural hearing loss. *Seminars in Perinatology, 29*, 173–181.

Robbins, A. M., Renshaw, J. J., & Berry, S. W. (1991). Evaluating meaningful auditory integration in profoundly hearing-impaired children. *American Journal of Otology, 12*(Suppl), 144–150.

Roberts, C., & Hindley, P. (1999). Practitioner review: the assessment and treatment of deaf children with psychiatric disorders. *Journal of Child Psychology and Psychiatry, 40*(2), 151–167.

Roeser, R., & Clark, J. (2008). Live voice speech recognition audiometry: Stop the madness. *Audiology Today, 20*, 32–33.

Roizen, N. J., Wolters, C., Nicol, T., & Blondis, T. A. (1993). Hearing loss in children with Down syndrome. *Journal of Pediatrics, 123*, S9–S12.

Rossi, K. (2003). *Talk around the clock.* Washington, DC: The Alexander Graham Bell Association for Deaf and Hard of Hearing.

Sanders, D. (1965) Noise conditions in normal school classrooms. *Exceptional Child, 31*, 344–353.

Scollie, S., Seewald, R., Cornelisse, L., Moodie, S., Bagatto, M., Laurnagaray, D., et al. (2005). The desired sensation level multistage input/output algorithm. *Trends in Amplification, 9*(4), 159–197.

Seewald, R. C., Ross, M., & Spiro, M. K. (1985). Selecting amplification characteristics for young hearing-impaired children. *Ear and Hearing, 6*, 48–51.

Seymour, F. K., Cruise, A., Lavy, J. A., Bradley, J., Beale, T., Graham, J. M., et al. (2010). Cognenital profound hearing loss: Management of hypoplastic and aplastic vestibulocochlear nerves. *Cochlear Implants International, 11*(Suppl 1), 213–216.

Shallop, J. K., Peterson, A., Facer, G. W., Fabry, L. B., & Driscoll, C. L. W. (2001) Cochlear implants in five cases of auditory neuropathy: Postoperative findings and progress. *Laryngoscope, 111*, 555–562.

Sharma, A., & Dorman, M. F. (2006). Central auditory development in children with cochlear implants: Clinical implications. *Advances in Otorhinolaryngology, 64*, 66–88.

Sharma, A., Nash, A. A., & Dorman, M. (2009). Cortical development, plasticity and re-organization in children with cochlear implants. *Journal of Communication Disorders, 42*(4), 272–279.

Skarzynski, H., Lorens, A., Piotrowska, A., & Anderson, I. (2006). Partial deafness cochlear implantation provides benefit to a new population of individuals with hearing loss. *Acta Oto-Laryngologica, 126*, 934–940.

Skinner, M. W., Holden, L. K., Holden, T. A., Demorest, M. E., & Fourakis, M. S. (1997). Speech recognition at simulated soft, conversational, and raised-to-loud vocal efforts by adults with cochlear implants. *Journal of the Acoustical Society of America, 101*(6), 3766–3782.

Smith, J. H., Bale, J. F., & White, K. R. (2005). Sensorineural hearing loss in children. *Lancet, 365*, 879–890.

Spahr, A. J., & Dorman, M. F. (2004). Performance of subjects fit with the Advanced Bionics CII and Nucleus 3G cochlear implant devices. *Archives of Otolaryngology—Head & Neck Surgery, 130*, 624–628.

Stovall, D. (1982). *Teaching speech to hearing impaired infants and children.* Springfield, IL: Charles C. Thomas.

Stredler-Brown, A., & DeConde Johnson, C. (2003). *Functional auditory performance indicators: An integrated approach to auditory development.* Colorado Department of Education, Special Education Services Unit. Retrieved from http://www.cde.state.co.us/cdesped/SpecificDisability-Hearing.html

Szagun, G., & Stumper, B. (2012). Age or experience? The influence of age at implantation, social and linguistic environment on language development in children with cochlear implants. *Journal of Speech, Language, and Hearing Research,* Apr 5 [Epub ahead of print].

Teagle, H. F. B., Rousch, P. A., Woodard, J. S., Hatch, D. R., Zdanski, C. J., Buss, E., et al. (2010). Cochlear implantation in children with auditory neuropathy spectrum disorder. *Ear and Hearing, 31*, 325–335.

Van Deun, L., van Wieringer, A., Scherf, F., Doggouj, N., Desloovere, C., Offeciers, F. E., et al. (2010). Earlier intervention leads to better sound localization in children with bilateral cochlear implants. *Audiology & Neurotology, 15*, 7–17.

Vescan, A., Parnes, L. S., Cucci, R. A., Smith, R. J., & MacNeill, C. (2002). Cochlear implantation and Pendred's syndrome mutation in monozygotic twins with large vestibular aqueduct syndrome. *Journal of Otolaryngology, 31*, 54–57.

Wackym, P. A., Runge-Samuelson, C. L., Firszt, J. B., Alkaf, F. M., & Burg, L. S. (2007). More challenging speech perception tasks demonstrate binaural benefit in bilateral cochlear implant users. *Ear and Hearing, 28*, 80S–85S.

Weichbold, V., Tsiakpini, L., Coninx, F., & D'Haese, P. (2005). Development of a parent questionnaire for assessment of auditory behaviour of infants up to two years of age. *Laryngorhinootologie, 84*(5), 328–334.

White, K. R., Vohr, B. R., Meyer, S., Widen, J. E., Johnson, J. L., Gravel, J. S., et al. (2005). A multisite study to examine the efficacy of the Otoacoustic Emission/Automated Auditory Brainstem Response Newborn Hearing Screening Protocol: Research design and results of the study. *American Journal of Audiology, 14*, S186–S199.

Wilson, B. S., & Dorman, M. F. (2008a). Cochlear implants: A remarkable past and a brilliant future. *Hearing Research, 242*(1–2), 3–21.

Wilson, B. S., & Dorman, M. F. (2008b). Cochlear implants: Current designs and future possibilities. *Journal of Rehabilitation Research and Development, 45*, 695–730.

Wolfe, J., Baker, S., Caraway, T., Kasulis, H., Mears, A., Smith, J., et al. (2007). 1-year postactivation results for sequentially implanted bilateral cochlear implant users. *Otology & Neurotology, 28*, 589–596.

Zimmerman-Phillips, S., Robbins, A. M., & Osberger, M. J. (2000). Assessing cochlear implant benefit in very young children. *Annals of Otology, Rhinology and Laryngology Supplement, 185*, 42–43.

4

Role of the Speech-Language Pathologist in the Assessment of Pediatric Cochlear Implant Candidacy

Emily Lund

INTRODUCTION

In the preoperative cochlear implant candidacy process, teams must consider the ways hearing loss has affected a child's development; therefore, team members apart from the audiologist and surgeon play a crucial role in determining cochlear implant candidacy. Speech-language pathologists (SLPs), for example, have training necessary to assess a child's speech, language, and academic skills (American Speech-Language-Hearing Association, 2010). Assessments from SLPs can provide information about a candidate's current level of functioning and rate of development. Furthermore, the SLP may help provide insight into expected outcomes for a child once he or she has a cochlear implant; thus, information from a speech-language pathologist can help a team make an informed decision about a child's candidacy and provide possible expectations for a child post-implant.

Many assessments are available to measure a child's communication skills. To effectively administer and interpret those assessments, professionals must understand the purpose of the instrument and the skills it actually measures. This chapter provides a description of general principles of standardized assessment, along with descriptions of specific evaluation tools and metrics that are widely used by SLPs working with hearing-impaired children. In addition, this chapter discusses evaluation and therapy schedules necessary for children with hearing loss prior to cochlear implantation.

PRINCIPLES OF STANDARDIZED EVALUATION

Speech-language pathologists often use standardized assessments for evaluations. Standardized assessments are designed to be administered in the same way to all students. Generally, standardized assessments can be divided into two categories: norm-referenced assessments and criterion-referenced assessments. These types of assessments can serve very different purposes. A norm-referenced assessment instrument is designed to determine if a child's skills (speech, language, etc.) are delayed compared with a sample of his or her peers. Essentially, these assessments serve to answer the question: Is a child delayed, or is he or she functioning within the range of normal (McCauley & Swisher, 1984)? To answer this question, norm-referenced tests assess broad skill sets. Criterion-referenced assessments, on the other hand, help to answer the question: Is a child able to perform a given skill/task to a certain criterion level? The criterion-referenced assessment does not compare a child with his or her peers but rather is based on the theory that a child should have mastered a set of skills by a given age and assesses the child's mastery of those skills (Swaminathan, Hambleton, & Algina, 1974). Criterion-referenced tests tend to assess specific skill sets. Understanding the difference between information derived from a norm-referenced versus criterion-referenced assessment is critical for interpretation of results.

Norm-Referenced Assessments

Norm-referenced assessments are designed to identify delayed skill sets, not to capture change over short periods of time. Specific items on norm-referenced assessments are included as a part of the instrument because they reliably distinguish between delayed versus typically developing children. These items are not thought to be representative of a child's performance across the entire range of a given skill. For example, the Clinical Evaluation of Language Fundamentals (fourth edition) assessment "Concepts and Following Direction" subtest has an item requiring children to "point to the shoe before [they] point to the houses" (Semel, Wiig, & Secord, 2003). A child's inability to complete this task does not indicate that he or she does not understand concepts or how to follow directions, nor does it indicate that a child who can answer this question has adequate auditory comprehension skills. Rather, this

item was chosen because, in combination with the other items on this instrument, performance on the item reliably separates children who do and do not have typical auditory comprehension skills; thus, performance on individual items from a norm-referenced assessment should not be used to discuss individual skill sets of a child, but only to talk broadly about whether a child is delayed or not.

Criterion-Referenced Assessments

Criterion-referenced assessments are designed to measure mastery of certain skill sets without reference to the performance of other children (Popham & Husek, 1969). These assessments often contain items ordered by level of difficulty. A child's performance on a criterion-referenced item or group of items should indicate mastery of a set of skills (Popham & Husek, 1969). For example, the PALS-PreK Letter Naming subtest requires children to identify the names of letters of the alphabet (Invernizzi, Sullivan, Meier, & Swank, 2004). If a child is unable to name specific letters, an examiner can conclude that the child's performance is indicative of his or her letter-naming skills. Because criterion-referenced assessments are designed to capture a child's mastery of a skill, they can be used to monitor progress.

ASSESSING CHILDREN WITH HEARING LOSS

An SLP involved in the cochlear implant candidacy process is charged with determining a child's current level of communicative functioning and potential outcomes post-implantation; thus, the SLP needs to be able to analyze a specific assessment's validity for measuring the skills of an individual child with hearing loss. Central to this task lies the question: Does the instrument capture a child's skill proficiency or ability? Proficiency is a child's skill level in comparison to a fluent adult model (Bachman & Savignon, 2002). Ability, on the other hand, is a child's capacity or potential to acquire skills (McNamara, 1995). This distinction between proficiency and ability in children with hearing loss is an important one during assessment interpretation, and subsequently for cochlear implant candidacy decisions and counseling.

Proficiency can be impacted by a child's environment; he or she may not display certain behaviors due to lack of opportunities to learn, not lack of ability. In addition to a child not being able to perform a skill because of his or her hearing status, the proficiency of the child may be also impacted by factors such as the socioeconomic status of his or her home environment. The ability to label objects, for example, may be impacted by a child's actual knowledge of the name of that object but may also be influenced by his or her family's experience with naming objects or with those specific objects at home (Lidz & Pena, 1996). Some cultures do not regularly label objects. Consequently, in a testing situation a child's deficient object labeling may not be representative of a lack of skill but rather reduced procedure familiarity.

A child's environment should not impact his or her innate ability or inability to acquire a skill (McNamara, 1995). For example, a child who lacks the ability to use the social rules of language may not be able to do so even when environmental factors (i.e., lack of familiarity with procedure) are improved; thus, a child's abilities may be predictive of his or her performance following implantation. Unfortunately, ability separate from environmental influence is difficult to measure (McNamara, 1995). Proficiency, change over time, and learning tasks often are used as indicators of a child's underlying ability (Lidz & Pena, 1996).

Speech-language pathologists working with children with hearing loss should have an understanding of specific assessments and whether they tap a child's ability or proficiency. Many assessments used with children, norm referenced or criterion referenced, were not specifically designed to address the needs of children with hearing loss. As a result, professionals who administer and interpret standardized assessments for children with hearing loss should be able to analyze the actual skills measured by the instrument. For example, many standardized assessments do not allow the examiner to repeat items to a child; thus, a child with hearing loss may miss an item measuring a language skill not because the child lacks that skill, but because he or she did not hear the question the first time. In this case, the assessment is not measuring a child's real language proficiency, but rather his or her ability to hear the question. This instrument, therefore, may be representative of a child's question-answering proficiency in a testing environment, but not his or her language proficiency or ability (i.e., answering questions within daily activities). For every assessment tool used to evaluate a child with hearing loss, a professional must consider the skill actually being assessed in relation to the conclusions he or she draws.

In the following sections, specific common assessment instruments for children with hearing loss are described to assist professionals in determining the utility of information presented for implant candidacy.

Specific Assessments

Assessments of Speech Production

Assessments of speech production, or articulation, are used to evaluate a child's phonological development, a key domain of oral language (Table 4–1). Patterns of speech production are observable and predictable even before children begin to use language. Vocalization and babble can provide valuable information about a child's articulatory development and possibly present red flags for delayed development (Robbins, 2005). Children with hearing loss have delayed early babbling behaviors, which may function as a precursor to their later speech delays (Moeller et al., 2007). Accordingly, careful characterization of a child's speech skills serves to demonstrate that a child is or is not developing appropriate precursor skills to good speech patterns, an important consideration in the cochlear implant candidacy process.

Because examiners cannot directly elicit infant speech patterns, most evaluation data at this age come from direct observation and parental reports. Many SLPs use articulation inventories or lists of phonemes a child may produce (standardized or not) to determine whether a child's vocalizations are developing at an expected rate. For example, SLPs know that children who are typically developing are expected to produce canonical babble

Table 4–1. Speech Production Assessment Instrument Reference Chart

Measure Name	Type of Measure	Domains Assessed	Age Range	Information Collected
Rosetti Infant–Toddler Language Scales (RI-TLS)	Criterion referenced	Subtests: interaction–attachment, pragmatics, gesture, play, language comprehension, language expression	0–36 months	Direct observation, behavior elicitation, parental report
Cottage Acquisition Scales for Listening, Language and Speech (CASSLS)	Criterion referenced	Forms available: pre-verbal, pre-sentence, simple sentence, complex sentence, sounds and speech	0–8 years	Direct observation, behavior elicitation, parental report
St. Gabriel's Curriculum for the Development of Audition, Language, Speech, and Cognition	Criterion referenced	Audition, speech, cognition, social interaction, fine motor skills, gross motor skills	0–6 years	Direct observation, behavior elicitation, parental report
Goldman-Fristoe Test of Articulation-2 (GFTA-2)	Norm referenced	Articulation	2–21 years	Behavior elicitation
Khan-Lewis Phonological Analysis, Second Edition (KLPA-2)	Criterion referenced (to be used in combination with GFTA-2)	Phonological processes (articulation)	2–21 years	Behavior elicitation
Arizona Articulation Proficiency Scale, Third Edition (AAPS-3)	Norm referenced	Articulation	1.5–18 years	Behavior elicitation

by the age of 10 months (Oller & Eilers, 1988). This benchmark may serve as an indicator to a professional that an infant's speech is or is not developing at the expected rate; however, speech patterns this early in development are broadly variable and should be interpreted as such.

Criterion-referenced checklists that evaluate speech production, along with several domains of behavior, can be useful for children with hearing loss. Many developmental scales use the principles of criterion-referenced instruments. The Rosetti Infant–Toddler Language Scale (RI-TLS) (Rossetti, 1990) is one example of a developmental scale used to measure language development, including speech production. This instrument requires an examiner to observe and elicit behavior, as well as solicit parental reports to determine whether a child possesses age-appropriate communicative skills. Behaviors on this scale are divided into the following domains: interaction–attachment, pragmatics, gesture, play, language comprehension, and language expression. Mastery within a domain is established when a child displays all of the behaviors within a given age range (e.g., 21–24 months); thus, delays are calculated as a percentage of a child's chronologic age. For example, a child with skills at 9–12 months who is 18 months old displays a 33% delay according to the RI-TLS.

Criterion-referenced instruments measuring multiple domains can help a cochlear implant team determine whether a child's speech-production development is consistent with his or her other skills. For example, a child with no delay in play skills but a 33% delay in speech-production skills clearly has a language-specific delay not predicted by his or her other skill proficiency. This result indicates that the access to sound that a child has is not sufficient for normal receptive language development. Other instruments used in a similar fashion to evaluate the speech production of infants and toddlers with hearing loss include the Cottage Acquisition Scales for Listening, Language and Speech (Wilkes, 1999) and St. Gabriel's Curriculum for the Development of Audition, Language, Speech, and Cognition (Tuohy, Brown, & Mercer-Moseley, 2005).

Speech-production patterns of typical preschool children are also highly variable. Articulation errors are still common at this age; however, patterns of error remain fairly predictable, and a child's errors that fall outside of these patterns (atypical errors) are less likely to correct naturally over time (Ohde & Sharf, 1992). A thorough evaluation of a preschool child's articulation and consequent intelligibility can provide a cochlear implant team with important information about a child's speech perception and possibly continued development (Eisenberg, 2007).

Speech-language pathologists have a broader range of instruments to choose from for preschool and school-age children because these children are able to produce and imitate words and sentences. The Goldman-Fristoe Test of Articulation-2 (GFTA-2), for example, is a norm-referenced test that requires children to produce single words in isolation or in sentences (preferably spontaneously) (Goldman & Fristoe, 2000). Each consonant in the English language is produced in word-initial, word-medial, and word-final positions. The number of errors tells an SLP whether or not the child's general articulation skills are age appropriate. As with other norm-referenced assessments, this instrument describes whether a child's articulation proficiency is within the range of normal for his or her age.

The GFTA-2 can be used in conjunction with the Khan-Lewis Phonological Analysis (KLPA-2) to describe a child's production error patterns (Khan & Lewis, 2002). This instrument identifies error patterns (i.e., backing, final-consonant deletion) based on a child's performance on the GFTA-2. Together, data from these instruments can be valuable to a cochlear implant team in determining whether a child's articulation is age appropriate and whether a child's patterns of articulation appear typical or atypical. In other words, a child who does not appear to have typical patterns of articulation may be a candidate for a cochlear implant because he or she is not developing speech-production skills appropriately.

The Arizona Articulation Proficiency Scale (AAPS-3) is another widely used, norm-referenced articulation assessment (Fudala, 2000). Like the GFTA-2, the AAPS-3 requires children to produce single words to label pictures. The AAPS-3 measures both consonant and vowel production; however, it does not measure each of the English consonants in different word-placement positions. Vowels are among the earliest produced sounds by children, and most children master vowel sounds before they master consonant sound production (Ohde & Sharf, 1992). Children with hearing loss, on the contrary, frequently display prolonged difficulty producing correct and consistent vowel sounds (Eisenberg, 2007). Consequently, the AAPS can provide valuable information to a cochlear implant team about a child's proficiency producing vowel sounds.

Assessments of Language

Language assessments can evaluate many domains of children's development, including vocabulary, grammar, and pragmatics. Prior to implantation, a team should have an understanding of how hearing loss has affected that child's ability to develop language. Many criterion-referenced and norm-referenced assessments are available to SLPs to evaluate both early and late stages of language development. Several common assessments of each type are described below. These descriptions, however, are not all encompassing; many additional assessments of language exist.

As with assessments of speech production, language assessments used with infants are primarily criterion referenced and based on parental reports or direct observation. One common criterion-referenced assessment of infant and toddler vocabulary is the MacArthur-Bates Communicative Development Inventory (Fenson et al., 2006). This instrument is based on parental reports; parents are asked to identify words, gestures, and phrases from daily life that a child is able to understand or produce. Instruments such as the CDI are useful for evaluating patterns of vocabulary knowledge and comparing a child's total number of vocabulary words to the number of words expected for his or her age. This information can demonstrate to a cochlear implant team that a child is or is not developing early vocabulary at an expected rate.

Common norm-referenced assessments of expressive and receptive vocabulary include the Peabody Picture Vocabulary Test (PPVT-4), The Expressive Vocabulary Test (EVT-2), the Receptive One Word Picture Vocabulary Test (ROWPVT-4), and the Expressive One Word Picture Vocabulary Test (EOWPVT-4) (Dunn & Dunn, 2006; Williams, 2007; Martin & Brownell, 2010a, 2010b). Receptive assessments (PPVT-4 and ROWPVT-4) require children to point to one of four pictures best represented by the examiner's label, whereas expressive assessments (EVT-2 and EOWPVT-4) require children to label a picture or group of pictures. A raw score is derived based on the number of correctly labeled or identified pictures and then compared with the scores of a child's same-age peers. These instruments are useful for determining whether or not a child has delayed vocabulary skills; however, these types of assessments do not describe a child's depth of vocabulary knowledge, nor do they represent patterns of knowledge (i.e., knows many individual labels but not superordinate category labels).

Many SLPs choose to use omnibus assessments of language development, especially as children begin to acquire grammar. Norm-referenced assessments for preschool-aged children include the Clinical Evaluation of Language Fundamentals (preschool edition), the Reynell Developmental Language Scales, the Receptive–Expressive Emergent Language Test (third edition), and the Preschool Language Scale (fifth edition), as well as many others (Semel, Wiig, & Secord, 2004; Reynell & Gruber, 1990; Bzoch & League, 1991; Zimmerman, Steiner, & Pond, 2010). These instruments assess a variety of domains (Table 4–2), requiring children to complete tasks such as following directions, identifying pictures, completing sentences, and answering questions. These instruments then yield subtest and total language

scores that a professional can compare with those of children of that child's same age. As with other norm-referenced assessments, these instruments do not reveal patterns of language errors because they only sample a few specific behaviors. Subtest scores, in fact, should be interpreted carefully; individual subtests may not share the overall sensitivity and specificity characteristics of a given instrument (Plante & Vance, 1995). Data from these assessments, however, can demonstrate to a cochlear implant team that a child has not developed language skills consistent with age expectations.

Some SLPs may also choose to administer criterion-referenced, omnibus assessments of language. The RI-TLS, for example, yields information about receptive and expressive language development. Many SLPs who work with children with hearing loss use scales specifically designed for children with hearing loss. For example, the Cottage Acquisition Scales for Listening, Language, and Speech (Wilkes, 1999) include checklists of skills within various domains, including listening comprehension, vocabulary, and grammatical development. Checklists represent various levels of language development, including pre-verbal, pre-sentence, simple sentence, and complex sentence levels. Similarly, the SKI-HI Language Development Scale (Watkins, 1979) provides parent and professional checklists of developmentally ordered receptive and expressive language skills. SLPs can determine, based on structured observation, whether or not a child has mastered those skills expected for his or her age. An advantage of these instruments is that they provide detailed examinations of specific language skills.

Assessments available to school-age children often assess higher-level language skills, such as making inferences or explaining word meanings. Information taken from these assessment instruments may be useful to cochlear implant teams evaluating the candidacy of an older child, such as one with a progressive loss. Some omnibus, norm-referenced language assessments for school-age children include the Clinical Evaluation of Language Fundamentals-Fourth Edition (Semel, Wiig, & Secord, 2003), the Oral and Written Language Scales (second edition) (Carrow-Woolfolk, 1995)

Table 4–2. Language Assessment Instrument Reference Chart

Measure Name	Type of Measure	Domains Assessed	Age Range	Information Collected
MacArthur-Bates Communicative Development Inventory (CDI)	Criterion referenced	Forms: words and gestures, words and sentences	8–30 months	Direct observation, parental report
Peabody Picture Vocabulary Test, Fourth Edition (PPVT-4)	Norm referenced	Receptive vocabulary	2.5–90 years	Behavior elicitation
Receptive One Word Picture Vocabulary Test, Fourth Edition (ROWPVT-4)	Norm referenced	Receptive vocabulary	2–18 years	Behavior elicitation
Expressive Vocabulary Test, Second Edition (EVT-2)	Norm referenced	Expressive vocabulary	2.5–90 years	Behavior elicitation
Expressive One Word Picture Vocabulary Test (EOWPVT-4)	Norm referenced	Expressive vocabulary	2–18 years	Behavior elicitation
Clinical Evaluation of Language Fundamentals, Preschool Edition (CELF-P)	Norm referenced	Composite scores: core language, receptive language, expressive language, language content, language structure	3–6 years	Behavior elicitation
Reynell Developmental Language Scales (RDLS)	Norm referenced	Receptive language, expressive language	1–6 years	Behavior elicitation
Receptive Expressive Emergent Language Test, Second Edition (REEL-3)	Norm referenced	Receptive language, expressive language	0–3 years	Parental report
Preschool Language Scale, Fifth Edition (PLS-5)	Norm referenced	Subtests: auditory comprehension, expressive language	0–6 years	Direct observation, behavior elicitation, parental report
Rosetti Infant–Toddler Language Scales (RI-TLS)	Criterion referenced	Subtests: interaction–attachment, pragmatics, gesture, play, language comprehension, language expression	0–36 months	Direct observation, behavior elicitation, parental report
Cottage Acquisition Scales for Listening, Language and Speech (CASSLS)	Criterion referenced	Forms available: pre-verbal, pre-sentence, simple sentence, complex sentence, sounds and speech	0–8 years	Direct observation, behavior elicitation, parental report

continues

Table 4–2. *continued*

Measure Name	Type of Measure	Domains Assessed	Age Range	Information Collected
St. Gabriel's Curriculum for the Development of Audition, Language, Speech, and Cognition	Criterion referenced	Audition, speech, cognition, social interaction, fine motor skills, gross motor skills	0–6 years	Direct observation, behavior elicitation, parental report
SKI-HI Language Development Scale	Criterion referenced	Receptive language, expressive language	0–5 years	Parental report
Clinical Evaluation of Language Fundamentals, Fourth Edition (CELF-4)	Norm referenced	Composite scores: core language, receptive language, expressive language, language content, language memory, working memory	5–21 years	Behavior elicitation
Oral and Written Language Scales (OWLS)	Norm referenced	Scales: listening comprehension, oral expression, written expression	3–21 years	Behavior elicitation
Comprehensive Assessment of Spoken Language (CASL)	Norm referenced	Receptive language, expressive language	3–21 years	Behavior elicitation
Test of Pragmatic Language, Second Edition (TOPL-2)	Norm referenced	Pragmatic language	6–18 years	Behavior elicitation
Test of Auditory Comprehension of Language, Third Edition (TACL-3)	Norm referenced	Receptive language	3–9 years	Behavior elicitation
The Word Test: Adolescents	Norm referenced	Vocabulary	≥12 years	Behavior elicitation
The Word Test: Elementary	Norm referenced	Vocabulary	6–11 years	Behavior elicitation

and the Comprehensive Assessment of Spoken Language (see Table 4–2) (Carrow-Woolfolk, 1999). These assessments require children to use their language skills to complete tasks such as comprehending paragraphs, following directions, and generating sentences. These instruments, like other norm-referenced assessments, yield general standard scores to compare a child's language skills with those of other children of the same age.

Because language deficits of school-age children may be subtle or limited to a certain language domain, many assessments target more specific language skills. The Test of Pragmatic Language (second edition) (Phelps-Terasaki & Phelps-Gunn, 1992), for example, rather than testing grammar or vocabulary knowledge, specifically assesses a child's ability to use language socially. The Test of Auditory Comprehension of Language (third edition) (Carrow-Woolfolk, 1998) assesses auditory comprehension skills but not expressive language. The Word Test (Bowers, Huisingh, LoGiudice, & Orman, 2005) taps semantic knowledge and organization by requiring children, for example, to name categories, generate synonyms, and name category members. Each of these instruments can provide information about deficits related to hearing loss that cause a child to continue to struggle academically. Such information is valuable to the cochlear implant team as they consider barriers to achieving language-skill proficiency.

Assessments of Auditory Skills

Evaluation of a child's candidacy for a cochlear implant should include assessments of his or her use of limited auditory skills in real-world situations (Table 4–3). An SLP can observe and assess the auditory behaviors of children over the course of a few visits. Auditory assessments can help a team determine whether a child's auditory behaviors are consistent with his or her responses to speech sounds in the audiology booth.

The Early Speech Perception Test (ESP) (Moog & Geers, 1990) is a criterion-referenced assessment instrument used by professionals to evaluate a child's ability to discriminate different types of sounds. A child is asked to differentiate between sounds of differing gross durations ("aaa" versus "hop hop hop"), between words of differing duration ("birthday cake" versus "bird"), and between words of the same duration with different phonemes ("bed" versus "book"). Young children can choose toys to match target words, and older children can point to pictures to demonstrate their discrimination skills. Benchmarks set by the authors (e.g., 8 of 12 correct responses) help professionals to determine whether a child has mastered the different levels of auditory discrimination.

The Auditory Perception Test for the Hearing Impaired, Revised (APT/HI-R) (Allen & Serwatka, 2008) is another criterion-referenced instrument appropriate for school-age children. This instrument requires children to complete a series of receptive tasks of varying difficulty, including discriminating between sounds differing in suprasegmental features, between words with differing syllable numbers or consonants, and between sentences containing different words. The demands of this instrument (pointing to pictures in a booklet) are similar to the demands of other standardized tasks children are asked to complete; thus, a child's performance on the APT/HI-R or the ESP

Table 4–3. Auditory Functioning Assessment Instrument Reference Chart

Measure Name	Type of Measure	Domains Assessed	Age Range	Information Collected
Early Speech Perception Test (ESP)	Criterion referenced	Auditory discrimination and identification	3–12 years	Behavior elicitation
Auditory Perception Test for the Hearing Impaired, Revised (APT/HI-R)	Criterion referenced	Auditory discrimination and identification	≥5 years	Behavior elicitation
Cottage Acquisition Scales for Listening, Language and Speech (CASSLS)	Criterion referenced	Forms available: preverbal, pre-sentence, simple sentence, complex sentence, sounds and speech	0–8 years	Direct observation, behavior elicitation, parental report
St. Gabriel's Curriculum for the Development of Audition, Language, Speech, and Cognition	Criterion referenced	Audition, speech, cognition, social interaction, fine motor skills, gross motor skills	0–6 years	Direct observation, behavior elicitation, parental report

may help an SLP to determine whether a child performs poorly on these instruments due limited auditory skills, limited language proficiency, or a combination of the two.

The measurement of functional auditory responses is difficult to separate from measurement of vocabulary and language knowledge. Consequently, results from either of these instruments should be interpreted with caution. Both instruments require children to recognize that spoken words can be consistently paired with objects or pictures, and to recall which spoken words are paired with any given set of objects. For example, a child may be able to discriminate between a one-syllable word and a three-syllable word, but he or she may demonstrate difficulty selecting "bird" versus "ice cream cone." Errors on either the ESP or the APT/HI-R could be influenced by lack of vocabulary knowledge rather than auditory skills. The interpretation of these instruments should therefore be combined with parent and clinician observation to determine how a child uses audition in his or her daily life. It may be that higher levels of auditory skill cannot be artificially separated from language knowledge.

Assessments of Academic Skills

Children who are candidates for cochlear implants after entering preschool have often been exposed to academic skills, most of which are language based. A thorough analysis of a child's communicative proficiency prior to receiving a cochlear implant, therefore, should include an assessment of his or her academic knowledge. An evaluation of a child's mastery of these skills can provide information about a child's ability to learn in a classroom setting.

Reading and writing are academic skills that are closely linked to language proficiency. Assessments of early literacy skills can predict later reading and writing achievement (Storch & Whitehurst, 2002). Because literacy outcomes of children with hearing loss are notoriously poor, cochlear implant teams may want to consider the impact of hearing loss on a child's early literacy abilities. Two norm-referenced assessments of early literacy skills are the Test of Preschool Early Literacy

(TOPEL) (Lonigan, Wagner, & Torgesen, 2002) and the Comprehensive Test of Phonological Processing (CTOPP) (Wagner, Torgesen, & Rashotte, 1999). These assessments measure skills related to later literacy achievement, such as phonological awareness, phonological working memory, letter-sound identification, and print awareness. These instruments yield scores that allow professionals to compare a child to his or her same-age peers.

Many criterion-referenced assessments of literacy skills are also available. The Phonological Awareness Literacy Screening assessments (Pre-K, K, and grades 1, 2, and 3) (Invernizzi, Meier, Swank, & Juel, 2004) are useful measures of literacy skills that include phonological awareness, print awareness, and early decoding abilities. These instruments evaluate a child's ability to complete literacy-related tasks. For example, if a child entering kindergarten should be able to identify sounds corresponding to letters, the PALS-Pre-K letter-sound subtest could be administered to see which sounds a child knows and does not know. The results of this kind of measure demonstrate to a cochlear implant team whether a child has been able to acquire the knowledge necessary to continue achieving academically.

Other assessments of academic concept knowledge include the Boehm Test of Basic Concepts (third edition) (BTBC) (Boehm, 2000) and the Bracken School Readiness Assessment (third edition) (BSRA) (Bracken, 2007). The BTBC requires children to show knowledge of concepts (such as "missing" or "below") by pointing to parts of pictures. The results of this assessment, however, should be interpreted with caution for children with hearing loss. Picture representations of these concepts often highlight the correct response within the picture. For example, the picture for the target "different" shows one different picture among several identical other pictures. Children with hearing loss may consistently display understanding of the concept by responding to salient pictured cues (one "different" picture among many that are the same) rather than responding to a known vocabulary word (comprehension of the word "different"). The BSRA assesses content knowledge of colors, letters, numbers, sizes, and shapes based on receptive and expressive responses. Both assessments can be used effectively to measure the academic concept knowledge of young children with hearing loss.

Older children often participate in formal academic assessment, and results from these assessments can also be useful to a cochlear implant team. Norm-referenced assessments of reading and other academic concepts, such as the Woodcock Reading Mastery Test (third edition) (Woodcock, 1998) or the Woodcock Johnson Test of Achievement–III (Woodcock, McGrew, & Mather, 2001), allow teams to compare a child's performance with that of other children of his or her age. Both instruments contain several subtests (Table 4–4), allowing professionals to evaluate a child's performance across several academic domains. Information from these instruments indicates to a team whether a child is performing academically at the level expected of his or her same-grade/age peers with normal hearing.

General education teachers and teachers of the deaf who interact regularly with students also can provide valuable insight to a cochlear implant team. Teachers often set benchmarks and use criterion-referenced assessments to monitor progress. As a result, classroom teachers of older children can provide important perspectives: a child's rate of academic growth may indicate that he or she is able or unable to keep up with work presented to children of his or her same grade. The Screening Instrument for Targeting Educational Risk (SIFTER) is a rating scale teachers can use to compare a child's academics, attention, communication, classroom participation, and school behavior to those of other children in the classroom (Anderson, 1989). The cochlear implant team can use teacher reports across standardized assessments to determine if lack of access to sound contributes to that child's ability to perform academic tasks in the classroom.

Considerations for Special Populations

A cochlear implant team is charged with determining a child's current level of functioning and his or her potential for development with a cochlear implant. This goal becomes even more difficult in evaluations of children who are not considered part of "mainstream" culture. For example, children who are dialect speakers or children who are bilingual cannot be adequately evaluated by assessments of language developed for monolingual, mainstream dialect English-speaking children. A thorough assessment of a non-mainstream language user requires additional knowledge and consideration.

To measure the language proficiency and ability of these children, professionals have some options available, but many assessments require additional work and preparation. SLPs may be able to find assessments normed on those particular special populations. For example, the Expressive One Word Picture Vocabulary Test (Spanish Bilingual Edition) (Brownell, 2001) was normed on a group of bilingual Spanish/English-speaking children. Instruments with bilingual norms, however, are scarce currently and certainly not available for all groups of bilingual children. An SLP may also choose to evaluate a child using a criterion-referenced assessment. In this case, the SLP must determine whether or not that child should have mastered a given set of skills despite his or her language differences. Criterion-referenced assessments can be used descriptively, but of course, they should be interpreted with caution. Finally, SLPs may choose to use nonstandard methods, such as dynamic assessment, to measure growth in children from these populations. Only professionals with deep understanding of the implications of dynamic assessment procedures, which can include test-teach-retest paradigms and administration modifications, should interpret these results (Lidz & Pena, 1996).

Although many of these methods are imperfect and/or time intensive for measuring the language ability or proficiency of these groups of children, cochlear implant teams are still obligated to evaluate these children to the best of their ability. It is not appropriate to "wait" for a child to develop adequate proficiency in the dominant language. Rather, professionals should be familiar with both languages to which a child is exposed and critically evaluate a child's performance across both languages to determine whether or not a child needs additional access to sound.

Table 4–4. Academic Skill Assessment Instrument Chart

Measure Name	Type of Measure	Domains Assessed	Age/Grade Range	Information Collected
Test of Preschool Early Literacy (TOPEL)	Norm referenced	Print awareness, phonological awareness, oral vocabulary	3–5 years	Behavior elicitation
Comprehensive Test of Phonological Processing (CTOPP)	Norm referenced	Phonological awareness, phonological memory, rapid naming	5–24 years	Behavior elicitation
Phonological Awareness Literacy Screening Measures (PALS-PreK, PALS-K, PALS-1-3)	Criterion referenced	Name writing, Alphabet knowledge, beginning sound awareness, rhyme awareness, nursery rhyme knowledge, print and word awareness, letter sounds, spelling, word recognition, passage reading, comprehension, fluency	Preschool–3rd Grade	Behavior elicitation
Boehm Test of Basic Concepts, Third Edition (BTBC)	Norm referenced	Basic concept knowledge	Kindergarten–2nd Grade	Behavior elicitation
Bracken School Readiness Assessment, Third Edition (BSRA)	Criterion referenced	Color knowledge, letter knowledge, numbers/counting, comparison/size knowledge, shape knowledge	3–6 years	Behavior elicitation
Woodcock Reading Mastery Test, Third Edition (WRMT-3)	Norm referenced	Subtests: phonological awareness, listening comprehension, letter identification, word identification, rapid automatic naming, oral reading fluency, word attack, word comprehension, passage comprehension	4.5–79 years	Behavior elicitation
Woodcock-Johnson Test of Achievement- III (WJTA-III)	Norm referenced	Subtests: letter–word identification, reading fluency, passage comprehension, word attack, reading vocabulary, spelling, writing fluency, writing samples, editing, spelling of sounds, punctuation and capitalization, calculation, math fluency, applied problems,	2–90 years	Behavior elicitation

Table 4–4. *continued*

Measure Name	Type of Measure	Domains Assessed	Age/Grade Range	Information Collected
Woodcock-Johnson Test of Achievement- III (WJTA-III) *continued*		quantitative concepts, story retell, understanding directions, picture vocabulary, oral comprehension, sound awareness, academic knowledge		
Screening Instrument for Targeting Educational Risk (SIFTER)	Criterion referenced	Academics, attention, communication, participation, behavior	Preschool– School Age	Teacher report

PREIMPLANTATION THERAPY CONSIDERATIONS

Even prior to receiving a cochlear implant, speech-language therapy can be a useful tool both for the purposes of intervention and evaluation, despite the fact that a child may not have access to the full range of speech sounds. The following sections describe the purpose of therapy during preimplant period of a child's development.

Therapy Following Identification

Following identification of a child's hearing loss, many parents are unsure how best to communicate with their child. Research indicates that hearing parents of children with hearing loss do not interact with their children in the same way as parents of children with normal hearing (Spencer, Bodner-Johnson, & Gutfreund, 1992). As a result, children with hearing loss may have even fewer opportunities to experience typical interactions and communication than children with typical hearing, beyond those opportunities lost due to limited access to sound.

An SLP or other early-intervention professional can be particularly valuable to families during the period immediately following identification. During this period, the interventionist can serve at least two purposes: (a) to educate parents about the future development and obstacles for their child with hearing loss and to provide support, and (b) to help parents interact with their child, ensuring that opportunities to learn basic communication skills are maximized. Most children with hearing loss are born to parents with normal hearing (Mitchell & Karchmer, 2004). As a result, at the time of identification most parents have little to no knowledge about hearing loss or its impact on communication development. A therapist is in a prime position to help parents gradually make sense of the overwhelming amount of information with which they are presented. Additionally, even without focusing on spoken language, parents can help their children with hearing loss to learn early communication skills. Children with hearing loss can learn to respond to communicative attempts, to gesture to direct attention, and to use a variety other communication methods. Interventionists can guide parents through basic communicative routines with their child with hearing loss.

Therapy Following Hearing Aid Fitting

Children eligible to receive cochlear implants by definition do not gain sufficient benefit from hearing aids (Eisenberg, Kirk, Martinez, Ying, Miyamoto, 2004); however, even minimal residual access to sound from hearing aids can improve a child's communicative development. Basic awareness of the presence or absence of sound at any level is the first step toward developing auditory skills. An SLP can help parents work toward optimizing opportunities to connect sounds with objects and actions prior to cochlear implantation.

Drawing a child's attention to sounds in his or her environment is one of the earliest recommendations made to parents of children with hearing loss (Niparko, 2000). An SLP can help parents to recognize and draw their child's attention to sounds during everyday activities. Parents' ability to recognize and draw attention to different types of sound, such as continuous noises (i.e., a running dishwasher) or intermittent noises (i.e., a microwave beep) can assist a child's development of basic sound discrimination. These early activities set a precedent for drawing a child's attention to sound post-implantation.

Therapy Following Baseline Speech-Language Skill Evaluation

Following a child's initial speech-language evaluation, continued regular visits to an SLP allow the SLP to track the auditory, speech, and language development of a child. The SLP can provide information to a cochlear implant team about how access to sound or a lack of access to sound impacts an individual child's development. Progress monitoring, in addition to baseline data, informs a team's expectations and consequently future recommendations for a child.

Regular therapy visits prior to implantation set a precedent for ongoing therapeutic intervention post-implantation. Developing a good relationship with an SLP is important for both parents and children. These early therapy sessions can help families and SLPs to develop effective therapist–parent communication early. During this time, SLPs have the opportunity to discuss developmental principles and normal and deviant language learning. These discussions give parents early understanding of the principles that guide therapy following implantation. In addition, children learn to participate in play activities, both adult led and child led, and the therapist can begin to understand what motivates and does not motivate a child.

CONCLUSION

The speech-language pathologist plays a crucial role in determining cochlear implant candidacy. The SLP can make predictions about expected communication outcomes for a child once he or she has a cochlear implant. Given the individual linguistic profiles, auditory skills, and life experiences of children with hearing loss, the role of the SLP should go beyond simply reporting test scores and performances; instead, the SLP, as a member of the cochlear implant team, should provide a sufficiently individualized profile of the child's communicative strengths and needs for the team to make a well-informed decision as to this child's potential benefit of implantation.

REFERENCES

Allen, S. G., & Serwatka, T. S. (2008). *Auditory perception test for the hearing impaired* (Revised). San Diego, CA: Plural.

American Speech-Language-Hearing Association. (2010). *Knowledge and skills required for the practice of audiologic/aural rehabilitation.* Retrieved from http://www.asha.org/policy

Anderson, K. L. (1989). *Screening identification for targeting educational risk.* Denver, CO: The Educational Audiology Association.

Bachman, L., & Savignon, S. (2002). The evaluation of communicative language proficiency: A critique of the ACTFL oral interview. *Modern Language Journal, 70,* 380–390.

Boehm, A. E. (2000). *Boehm test of basic concepts* (3rd ed.). San Antonio, TX: The Psychological Corporation.

Bowers, L., Huisingh, R., LoGiudice, C., & Orman, J. (2005). *The word test–2: Adolescent.* Moline, IL: LinguiSystems.

Bracken, B. A. (2007). *Bracken school readiness assessment* (3rd ed.). San Antonio, TX: The Psychological Corporation.

Brownell, R. (2001). *Expressive one-word picture vocabulary test: Spanish-bilingual edition.* Novato, CA: Academic Therapy.

Bzoch, K., & League, R. (1991). *The Bzoch–League receptive and expressive emergent language test (REEL-2)* (2nd ed.). Austin, TX: Pro-Ed.

Carrow-Woolfolk, E. (1995). *Oral and written language scales (OWLS)*. Los Angeles, CA: Western Psychological Services.

Carrow-Woolfolk, E. (1998). *Test for auditory comprehension of language (TACL-3)* (3rd ed.). Austin, TX: Pro-Ed.

Carrow-Woolfolk, E. (1999). *Comprehensive assessment of spoken language (CASL)*. Los Angeles, CA: Western Psychological Services.

Dunn, L. A., & Dunn, L. M. (2006). *Peabody picture vocabulary test (PPVT-4)* (4th ed.). Circle Pines, MN: AGS.

Eisenberg, L. S. (2007). Current state of knowledge: Speech recognition and production in children with hearing impairment. *Ear and Hearing, 28*, 766–772.

Eisenberg, L. S., Kirk, K. E., Martinez, A. S., Ying, E. A., & Miyamoto, R. T. (2004). Communication abilities of children with aided residual hearing. *Archives of Otolaryngology—Head & Neck Surgery, 130*, 563–569.

Fenson, L., Marchman, V., Thal, D., Dale, P., Reznick, S., & Bates, E. (2006). *The MacArthur Communicative Development Inventories: User's guide and technical manual* (2nd ed.). Baltimore, MD: Brookes.

Fudala, J. B. (2000). *Arizona articulation proficiency scale (AAPS-3)* (3rd revision). Los Angeles, CA: Western Psychological Services.

Goldman, R., & Fristoe, M. (2000). *Goldman Fristoe test of articulation (GFTA-2)* (2nd ed.). Circle Pines, MN: AGS.

Invernizzi, M., Meier, J. D., Swank, L., & Juel, C. (2004). *PALS: Phonological awareness literacy screening*. Charlottesville, VA: University of Virginia Press.

Invernizzi, M., Sullivan, A., Meier, J., & Swank, L. (2004). *Phonological awareness literacy screening PreK (PALS-PreK)*. Charlottesville, VA: University of Virginia Press.

Khan, L., & Lewis, N. (2002). *Khan-Lewis phonological analysis* (2nd ed.). Circle Pines, MN: AGS.

Lidz, C., & Pena, E. (1996). Dynamic assessment: the model, its relevance as a nonbiased approach, and its application to Latino American preschool children. *Language, Speech, and Hearing Services in Schools, 27*, 367–372.

Lonigan, C. J., Wagner, R. K., & Torgesen, J. K. (2002). *Test of preschool early literacy (TOPEL)*. Austin, TX: Pro-Ed.

Martin, N. A., & Brownell, R. (2010a). *Expressive one word picture vocabulary test-4 (EOWPVT-4)*. Novato, CA: Academic Therapy.

Martin, N. A., & Brownell, R. (2010b). *Receptive one word picture vocabulary test-4. (ROWPVT-4)*. Novato, CA: Academic Therapy.

McCauley, R. J., & Swisher, L. (1984). Use and misuse of norm-referenced tests in clinical assessment: a hypo-thetical case. *Journal of Speech and Hearing Disorders, 49*, 338–348.

McNamara, T. K. (1995). Modeling performance: Opening Pandora's box. *Applied Linguistics, 16*, 159–179.

Mitchell, R. E., & Karchmer, M. A. (2004). Chasing the mythical ten percent: Parental hearing status of deaf and hard of hearing students in the United States. *Sign Language Studies, 4*, 138–163.

Moeller, M. P., Hoover, B., Putman, C., Arbataitis, K., Bohnenkamp, G., & Peterson, B., et al. (2007). Vocalizations of infants with hearing loss compared with infants with normal hearing, part I: Phonetic development. *Ear and Hearing, 28*, 605–627.

Moog, J. S., & Geers, A. (1990). *Early speech perception test for profoundly hearing-impaired children*. St. Louis, MO: Central Institute for the Deaf.

Niparko, J. (2000). *Cochlear implants: Principles and practices* (2nd ed.). Baltimore, MD: Lippincott, Williams and Wilkins.

Ohde, R. N., & Sharf, D. J. (1992). *Phonetic analysis of normal and abnormal speech*. New York, NY: Macmillan.

Oller, D. K., & Eilers, R. E. (1988). The role of audition in babbling. *Childhood Development, 59*, 441–449.

Phelps-Terasaki, D., & Phelps-Gunn, T. (1992). *Test of pragmatic language (TOPL-2)* (2nd ed.). Austin, TX: Pro-Ed.

Plante, E., & Vance, R. (1995). Diagnostic accuracy of two tests of preschool language. *American Journal of Speech and Language Pathology, 4*, 70–76.

Popham, W. J., & Husek, T. R. (1969). Implications of criterion referenced measurement. *Journal of Educational Measurement, 6*, 1–9.

Reynell, J. K., & Gruber, C. P. (1990). *Reynell developmental language scales*. Los Angeles, CA: Western Psychological Services.

Robbins, A. M. (2005). Clinical red flags for slow progress in children with cochlear implants. *Loud and Clear, 1*, 1-8.

Rossetti, L. (1990). *Rosetti Infant-Toddler Language Scale (RI-TLS)*. East Moline, IL: LinguiSystems.

Semel, E., Wiig, E. H., & Secord, W. A. (2003). *Clinical Evaluation of Language Fundamentals (CELF-4)* (4th ed.). San Antonio, TX: The Psychological Corporation.

Semel, E., Wiig, E., & Secord, W. A. (2004). *Clinical Evaluation of Language Fundamentals—Preschool (CELF-P2)* (2nd ed.). San Antonio, TX: The Psychological Corporation.

Spencer, P. E., Bodner-Johnson, B. A., & Gutfreund, M. K. (1992). Interaction with infants with hearing loss: What can we learn from mothers who are deaf? *Journal of Early Intervention, 16*, 64–78.

Storch, S. A., & Whitehurst, G. J. (2002). Oral language and code-related precursors to reading: Evidence from a longitudinal structural model. *Developmental Psychology, 38*, 934–947.

Swaminathan, H., Hambleton, R. K., & Algina, J. (1974). Reliability of criterion-referenced tests: A decision-theoretic formulation. *Journal of Educational Measurement, 11,* 264–267.

Tuohy, J., Brown, J., & Mercer-Moseley, C. (2005). *St. Gabriel's curriculum for the development of audition, language, speech, cognition, early communication, social interaction, fine motor skills, and gross motor skills* (2nd ed.). Sydney, Australia: St. Gabriel's Auditory-Verbal Early Intervention Centre.

Wagner, R. K., Torgesen, J., & Rashotte, C. (1999). *Comprehensive Test of Phonological Processing (CTOPP).* Austin, TX: Pro-Ed.

Watkins, S. (1979). *SKI-HI Language Development Scale.* Logan, UT: SKI-HI Institute.

Wilkes, E. M. (1999). *Cottage AcquisitionScales for Listening, Language, and Speech.* San Antonio, TX: Sunshine Cottage School for Deaf Children.

Williams, K. (2007). *Expressive Vocabulary Test (EVT-2)* (2nd ed.). Circle Pines, MN: AGS.

Woodcock, R. M. (1998). *Woodcock Reading Mastery Test* (revised). Circle Pines, MN: AGS.

Woodcock, R. W., McGrew, K. S., & Mather, N. (2001). *Woodcock–Johnson III test of achievement.* Itasca, IL: Riverside.

Zimmerman, I. L., Steiner, B. S., & Pond, R. E. (2010). *Preschool Language Scale (PLS-5)* (5th ed.). San Antonio, TX: The Psychological Corporation.

‖‖5‖‖

Nontraditional Candidates for Cochlear Implantation

René H. Gifford

INTRODUCTION

The FDA-labeled indications for adult and pediatric cochlear implant candidacy have remained unchanged for over 10 years. Medicare's National Coverage Determination outlining cochlear implantation criteria was last updated in July 2005. As stated in Chapter 1, in order for the implant manufacturers to broaden or expand the labeled indications (also referred to as candidacy criteria), they must complete an FDA-approved clinical trial requiring a panel-track supplement. This is a time intensive and extremely costly endeavor; thus, although technology and clinical practice has evolved rapidly over the past decade, the FDA-labeled indications remain unchanged.

Clinics across the country are routinely implanting patients who may not perfectly fit the implant candidate profile as specified in the labeled indications. The reason that this is occurring is that literature and clinical practice has provided us with evidence supporting the expansion of implant criteria.

This chapter describes the literature, current clinical practices, and the importance of evaluating the whole patient for the determination of implant candidacy for both adults and children.

BARRIERS TO COCHLEAR IMPLANTATION

As of December 2010, the FDA reported that approximately 43,000 adults and 28,000 children had received cochlear implants in the United States (NIH, 2011). That same year it had been reported that 34.25 million people in the United States had significant hearing difficulty (Kochkin, Beck, Christensen, Compton-Conley, Fligor, Kricos, et al., 2010). The NIDCD further estimates that up to 750,000 Americans have severe-to-profound hearing loss (NIDCD, 2010). Using 2010 census data, that would translate to over 11% of the U.S. population having *significant* hearing loss impacting communication; thus, with roughly 71,000 cochlear implant recipients in the United States as of 2010, less than 10% of the 750,000 individuals that could derive significant benefit from cochlear implants had actually been implanted. It is estimated that the underutilization of cochlear implant technology is mostly applicable to the adult populations, because it has been reported that 55% all pediatric implant candidates between the ages of 1 and 6 years actually get implanted (Bradham & Jones, 2008).

The underutilization of cochlear implant technology has many possible underlying sources. One possibility is the lack of patient awareness about cochlear implants. Cochlear implants have been referred to as the most successful sensory prosthesis invented (Wilson & Dorman, 2008). Given the success of cochlear implants and the ubiquity of related research in the peer-reviewed literature in otology, hearing, deaf education, speech, and language, one would assume that public awareness is also widespread. This, however, is not the case. The lack of widespread public awareness regarding cochlear implants, including function, candidacy, and insurance coverage, is a large part of the mission for a number of not-for-profit advocacy and awareness foundations including the American Cochlear Implant Alliance, Cochlear Implant Awareness Foundation, Hearing Loss Association of America, Alexander Graham Bell Association, Songs for Sound, the CARE project, Hearing Health Foundation, Hands and Voices, and others.

Another possible explanation for the underutilization of cochlear implants is a matter of finances. Stern, Yueh, Lewis, Norton, and Sie (2005) examined the ZIP codes of cochlear implant recipients, the associated median income in those codes, and found that more children living in higher socioeconomic areas had cochlear implants. This finding is cause for concern given that epidemiologic research has shown a greater prevalence of childhood hearing loss in lower socioeconomic areas (Mehra, Eavey, & Keamy, 2009). Finances also present a barrier to implant technology for adult candidates. There is an increasing trend for state Medicaid services to exclude cochlear implant coverage for individuals over 21 years of age. At the time of writing, the majority of states in the United States had instituted exclusions for cochlear implants in adults over 21 years in an effort to contain the growing costs of Medicaid services.

Another financial burden exists for individuals not meeting income requirements for Medicaid but whose employer does not offer health insurance coverage. According to the Centers for Disease Control, 46.3 million Americans of all ages were uninsured in 2011 (Cohen & Martinez, 2012). Those people who are uninsured may choose to forego health insurance coverage completely or purchase high-deductible health plans which may exclude cochlear implantation. Such exclusionary policies may only become problematic in cases of sudden or acquired adult hearing loss leaving the policyholder without cochlear implant coverage and lacking the finances to pay for the surgery, device, and external activation kit, all of which is estimated to cost between $45,000 and $120,000 depending on geographic location. The barrier to affordable insurance coverage, however, will likely be lessened with the passing of the Affordable Care Act in 2010.

Another barrier to implant technology may be related to the lack of professional knowledge among referring providers. This is not meant to solely implicate primary care physicians (Wu, Zardouz, Rothholtz, German, & Djalilian, 2010) and hearing aid dispensers (Huart & Sammeth, 2009) who may expectedly lack current knowledge about cochlear implant criteria. Even general ENT physicians and nonimplant audiologists may not fully recognize the audiologic profile of the modern-day implant candidate. Unless a professional has actively sought continuing education opportunities in the area of cochlear implant candidacy and outcomes, he or she may be under the impression that an individual must have profound bilateral deafness in order to qualify and derive benefit.

Yet another potential barrier to implantation relates to a lack of cochlear implant referrals from hearing aid dispensers and private-practice audiologists for fear of losing hearing aid patients. Though no data exist suggesting that hearing aid dispensers and/or private-practice audiologists are reluctant to refer for cochlear implant evaluation, it is not an unreasonable supposition. For professionals whose income relies either solely or predominantly upon hearing aid sales, a cochlear implant referral may be perceived as a lost patient; however, this is absolutely not the case. There are an increasing number of studies demonstrating that individuals making use of a cochlear implant and a contralateral hearing aid (also referred to as bimodal hearing) are able to integrate the electric and acoustic signals to derive significant benefit for speech recognition in quiet and in noise (e.g., Tyler, Parkinson, Wilson, Witt, Preece, & Noble, 2002; Mok, Grayden, Dowell, & Lawrence, 2006; Ching, van Wanrooy, & Dillon, 2007; Gifford, Dorman, McKarns, & Spahr, 2007; Dorman, Gifford, Lewis, McKarns, Ratigan, Spahr, et al., 2009) as well as for the recognition of music (e.g., Dorman et al., 2009; El Fata, James, Laborde, & Fraysee, 2009; Sucher & McDermott, 2009). The reality is that the bimodal listener can continue to be a unilateral hearing aid patient for many years and will respect the referring audiologist for knowing the limitations of hearing aids and recognizing when to appropriately refer for implant evaluation.

EVIDENCE FOR THE EXPANSION OF COCHLEAR IMPLANT CANDIDACY

Adults

A number of studies have reported speech understanding outcomes for adult implant recipients who had not met all FDA-labeled indications for cochlear implantation. Adunka, Buss, Clark, Pillsbury, and Buchman (2008) reported significant improvement in postoperative speech recognition abilities for 21 subjects with substantial residual hearing who had preoperative speech recognition of 72% for City University of New York (CUNY) sentences and 18% for consonant nucleus consonant (CNC) words. In addition, they demonstrated that the 21 non-traditional implant candidates had demonstrated equivalent benefit to a group of standard implant recipients, all of whom had met FDA-labeled indications for implantation. Furthermore, speech recognition improved for all participants in the study.

Tremblay et al. (2008) reported significant benefit for 17 implant recipients who had pre-implant sentence scores ranging from 40 to 77%. They reported a mean postoperative improvement of 38 percentage points for sentence recognition and 31 percentage points for word recognition. Speech understanding improved for all study participants.

Gifford et al. (2010) also reported significant benefit for 22 adult, nontraditional recipients whose preoperative speech recognition scores were 60% correct for Hearing in Noise Test (HINT) sentences, 47% for AzBio sentences, and 41% for CNC words. The mean postoperative improvement for CNC word recognition was 27 and 41 percentage points in the implant-only and best-aided conditions, respectively. Furthermore, speech understanding improved for all study participants.

Amoodi et al. (2011) reported significant postoperative improvement in speech recognition for 27 recipients who had scored 60% or greater for HINT sentence recognition preoperatively. The mean improvement for their subjects was 37 percentage points for CNC words and 27 percentage points for HINT sentences, though benefit from HINT sentence recognition was clearly limited by postoperative ceiling effects (see also Gifford, Shallop & Peterson, 2008). Speech understanding improved for all study participants.

Figure 5–1 summarizes the findings of the above-cited studies on nontraditional adult implant recipients. The degree of benefit averaged across all four studies was 38 percentage points for CNC word recognition and 33 percentage points for sentence recognition, though postoperative sentence recognition scores were limited by ceiling effects for many of the participants. Clearly the research on nontraditional adult implant recipients has been unequivocal in demonstrating improvement in speech perception. In fact, the point of diminishing returns has yet to be identified.

At the time of chapter preparation, Cochlear Americas had begun participant enrollment in an FDA-approved IDE study of revised indications for cochlear implantation (G090032/S005, 2011). The criterion for preoperative speech understanding for this clinical trial is CNC word recognition up to 40% in the ear to be implanted and no greater than 50% in the contralateral aided condition; thus, it is likely that adult cochlear implant criteria will be "officially" expanded in the near future. This path will continue to be investigated via evidence-based practices as we study the population who might benefit from cochlear implantation and, above all, strive to *do no harm*.

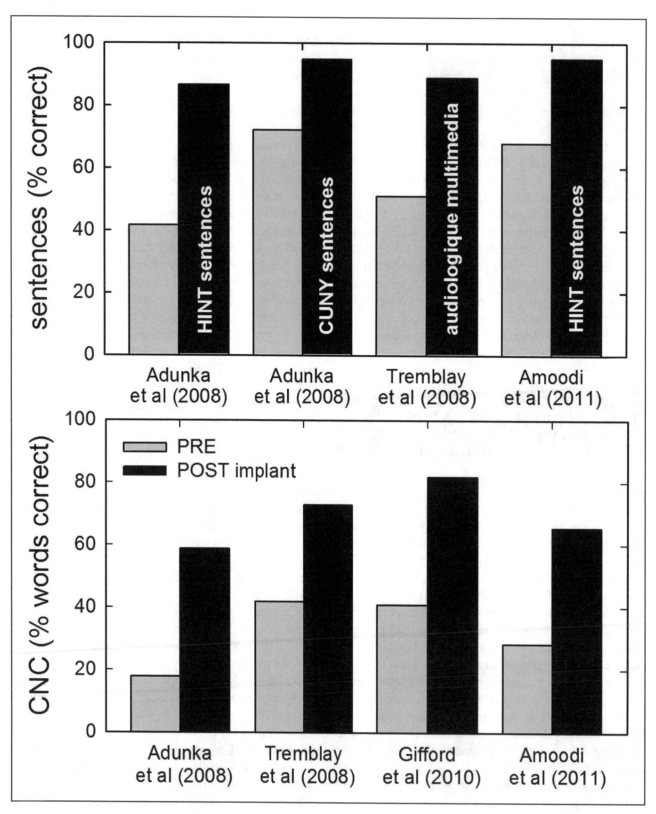

FIGURE 5–1. Comparison of pre- and postimplant consonant nucleus consonant (*CNC*) word recognition across studies specifically investigating the efficacy of cochlear implantation for adult candidates with significant residual hearing and/or above criterion preoperative speech recognition. **HINT** Hearing in Noise Test; **CUNY** City University of New York.

Children

Cochlear implant programs affiliated with large academic medical centers have been, for some time, routinely implanting children with sensory hearing loss who do not meet the "typical" implant candidacy profile. The reason that this is generally considered common practice is that evidence exists for the expansion of current implant criteria for children with significant hearing loss who are not making expected progress for auditory, speech, and language skills with appropriately fitted hearing aids and recommended intervention. Historically there have been a number of reports advocating for the expansion of pediatric cochlear implant criteria (e.g., Cowan, DelDot, Barker, Sarant, Pegg, Dettman, et al.,1997; Tomblin, Spencer, Flock, Tyler, & Gantz, 1999; Gantz, Rubinstein, Tyler, Teagle, Cohen, Waltzman, et al., 2000; Mondain, Sillon, Vieu, Levi, Reuillard-Artieres, Deguine, et al., 2002; Winton, Hollow, & Dettman, 2002; Eisenberg, Martinez, Holowecky, & Pogorelsky, 2002). There have been other reports of children with residual hearing successfully combining electric and acoustic stimulation across ears for bimodal hearing (e.g., Ching, Psarros, Hill, Dillon, & Incerti, 2001; Ching, Hill, Brew, Incerti, Priolo, Rushbrook, et al., 2005; Ching, Incerti, Hill, & van Wanrooy, 2006; Holt, Kirk, Eisenberg, Martinez, & Campbell, 2005; Beijen, Mylanus, Leeuw, & Snik, 2008; Straatman, Rietveld, Beijen, Mylanus, & Mens, 2010; Mok, Galvin, Dowell, & McKay, 2010); however, over the past decade there have only been a handful of peer-reviewed papers dealing specifically with the issue of expanded criteria for pediatric cochlear implantation.

Dettman, D'Costa, Dowell, Winton, Hill, and Williams (2004) evaluated pre- and post-implant performance for open-set speech recognition in a group of 16 children who had achieved preoperative sentence recognition scores above 30% correct. All but one of the study participants demonstrated significant improvement in word- and sentence-recognition performance. The one child who had exhibited a postoperative decrement in performance had only 6 months experience with the implant and his pre- and post-implant scores differed by less than 10 percentage points—a level that was not considered statistically significant at the single-subject level; thus, it is likely that over time this child's performance would have improved, or at best, would not have changed relative to pre-implant levels. It is important to note, however, that the children in this current study would have met FDA-labeled indications relative to degree of hearing loss because the mean pure tone average (PTA) was 109 and 96 dB HL for the implanted and non-implanted ears, respectively.

Yoshinago-Itano, Baca, and Sedey (2010) studied repeated measures of auditory–oral language growth for 87 children with severe-to-profound hearing loss who had either been fitted with hearing aids ($n = 38$) or cochlear implants ($n = 49$). The children had been followed over time and the trajectory of language growth was tracked up to 7 years. Their findings showed that children with cochlear implants exhibited a more rapid growth of receptive and expressive language than the children with hearing aids. Furthermore, they found that children with cochlear implants closed the language gap relative to age-equivalent peers with normal hearing. Children with hearing aids, however, closed the gap at a much slower pace for receptive language and did not close the gap for expressive language, at the group level; thus, these data could be interpreted as further evidence for expanding criteria to include at least severe hearing losses for the youngest candidates.

One of the most comprehensive studies examining expanded indications for pediatric cochlear implantation originates from Melbourne, Australia. Leigh, Dettman, Dowell, and Sarant (2011) evaluated speech recognition performance for 142 children with hearing loss who were either fitted with hearing aids ($n = 62$) or cochlear implants ($n = 80$). They reported that for children with a PTA greater than 60 dB HL, there is a 75% chance of improvement with a cochlear implant for word recognition performance. Using sentence recognition performance as a guide, a PTA greater than 72 dB HL would have a 75% chance for improvement with an implant; thus, they conservatively concluded that children with a PTA of 75 dB HL or greater should be recommended for cochlear implantation, at least unilaterally. Indeed one could interpret their findings to promote cochlear implantation for children with even less severe losses, provided that the child is not demonstrating *at least* year-for-year progress with speech, language, and auditory skills (see also Chapter 3).

Infants Under 12 Months of Age

As stated in Chapters 1 and 3, current labeled indications for pediatric candidacy list children 12 months of age and older. This age restriction is not to imply that infants under 12 months would not benefit from cochlear implantation. There is a growing body of literature demonstrating higher levels of word and language acquisition (Bergeson, Houston & Miyamoto, 2010; Houston & Miyamoto, 2010; Houston, Stewart, Moberly, Hollich, & Miyamoto, 2012; Niparko, Tobey, Thal, Eisenberg, Wang, Quittner, et al., 2010; Moog & Geers, 2010), speech perception (Tajudeen, Waltzman, Jethanamest, & Svirsky, 2010), speech-production intelligibility (Habib, Waltzman, Tajudeen, & Svirsky, 2010), and vocabulary development (Hayes, Geers, Treiman, & Moog, 2009; Houston & Miyamoto, 2010; Tomblin, Barker, Spencer, Zhang, & Gantz, 2005) for children implanted under 12 months of age, even when compared with children implanted in the second year of life.

One of the historical concerns about implanting infants under 12 months of age has been the issue of specificity—or the risk of implanting a child *without* permanent sensory hearing loss. With the audiologic tests at our disposal, including otoacoustic emissions, electrophysiologic measures, and advanced behavioral audiometric techniques for use in children as young as 5–6 months, initial diagnostic and then confirmatory diagnostic testing at very young ages is possible.

Cosetti and Roland (2010) explain that there is a wealth of literature on the surgical and anesthetic-related risks associated with surgery in infants. Specifically, there is a higher incidence of morbidity, mortality, and life-threatening adverse surgical events for children under 12 months who undergo surgery; however, Cosetti and Roland explain that the majority of concerns and complications reported in the literature have been confounded by emergency surgery for which there has been a lack of fasting and hence greater risk of aspiration, as well as the risks of surgery in healthy children and possibly medially fragile infant (under 1 month of age). As related to cochlear implant surgery, there are a number of studies demonstrating no greater anesthetic risk for infants under 12 months (James & Papsin, 2004; Colletti, Carner, Miorelli, Guida, Colletti & Fiorino, 2005; Miyamoto, Houston, & Bergeson, 2005; Miyamoto, Hay-McCutcheon, Kirk, Houston, & Bergeson-Dana, 2008; Waltzman & Roland, 2005; Dettman Pinder, Briggs, Dowell, & Leigh, 2007; Valencia, Rimell, Friedman, Oblander, & Helmbrecht, 2008). Cosetti and Roland outlined those surgical issues that are unique to infants under 12 months and those include intraoperative blood loss, facial nerve anatomy, skull thickness (<1 mm), fixation of the receiver/stimulator package, thin scalp flap, and device migration with skull growth. They reported, however, that these are known variables and can be mitigated with a highly trained surgical team having extensive pediatric experience.

Given the highly favorable risk/benefit ratio for implanting infants under 12 months, one might conclude that most children being identified at or near birth are routinely being implanted early. It is certainly the case that the request for insurance authorization is being submitted for infants as young as 6 to 9 months. The barrier to access for this population is that many insurance companies will often initially deny coverage citing that the FDA-labeled indications specify candidacy for children 12 months of age and older. There is a precedent for successful appeal particularly in peer-to-peer review when surgeons and audiologists are advocating for their patients; however, many state Medicaid programs deny authorization until a child reaches the 1-year mark. It may be the case that in the very near future a cost–utility study will promote cochlear implantation in children under 12 months given cost-saving measures (i.e., fewer hearing-related services) as the child ages.

UNILATERAL AND ASYMMETRIC HEARING LOSS

Implant candidacy has historically been based on speech recognition in the best-aided condition. To date, only one of the implant manufacturers has even made reference to considering preoperative performance in the ear to be implanted in their labeled indications for adult candidates (Cochlear Americas physicians package insert). The prevalence of asymmetric hearing loss among sensorineural losses is estimated at 50–57% (Margolis & Saly, 2008; Liu et al., 2011); hence, it is reasonable to presume that the "best-aided condition" may overestimate one's hearing and speech understanding, particularly for realistic listening environments in which the target stimulus may not always be directed toward the front or the better-hearing ear.

As mentioned in Chapter 3, the revised Minimum Speech Test Battery (MSTB, 2011) recommends individual ear assessment of speech-understanding performance. This recommendation raises the question of whether we should be determining implant candidacy on the basis of the *ear to be implanted*. Firszt, Holden, Reeder, Cowdrey, and King (2012) described the outcomes for ten adult recipients with asymmetric hearing loss for which implant candidacy was determined on the basis of the poorer-hearing ear. In the non-implanted ear, four of the ten subjects had low-frequency audiometric thresholds in the normal to near-normal range. Even with the highly asymmetric nature of the hearing losses in their population, they showed significant improvement in speech recognition performance in quiet and noise as well as localization abilities. These findings suggest that we should consider implant candidacy on an individual-ear basis even when the better-hearing ear exceeds traditional candidacy criteria. Firszt and colleagues noted, however, that adults with pre- or peri-lingual onset of deafness in the poorer-hearing ear achieved modest benefit and thus may require more extensive preoperative counseling regarding realistic expectations.

Other cases of cochlear implantation with asymmetric hearing loss have focused on tinnitus suppression rather than improving speech recognition. There are multiple reports of the benefits of cochlear implantation for patients with unilateral hearing loss as a means for tinnitus suppression (van de Heyning et al., 2008; Kleinjung, Steffens, Strutz, & Langguth, 2009; Vermeire & van de Heyning, 2009; Buechner et al., 2010; Punte et al., 2011; Amoodi et al., 2011; Arndt, Aschendorff, Laszig, Beck, Schild, Kroeger, Ihorst, & Wesarg, 2011; Ramos et al., 2012). Thus far, the majority

of reports describing cochlear implantation for tinnitus relief in cases of unilateral hearing loss have resulted in positive outcomes. In some cases, there were even reports of improved speech recognition in noise and subjective reports of hearing benefit (Buechner et al., 2010; Arndt et al., 2011). All reports of cochlear implants for tinnitus relief in cases of unilateral hearing loss have originated from European centers and most were implanted under the umbrella of a clinical trial. Despite the increased interest in this topic in recent years, it remains unclear whether cochlear implantation for tinnitus suppression in cases of unilateral hearing loss is a cost efficient and viable treatment option and whether this is a treatment that would be covered by insurance as a medical necessity.

PRELINGUALLY DEAFENED ADOLESCENTS AND ADULTS

When multichannel cochlear implants were first granted FDA approval for adults in 1985, the criteria specified that candidates must have postlingual onset of hearing loss. The concern was that the auditory centers of the brain would be unable to make use of the new electric stimulus, and thus outcomes for speech understanding would be poor. Some of the pioneering researchers in the field published reports of relatively small samples of prelingually deafened adults who had received cochlear implants (Hinderink, Snik, Mens, Brokx, & Van den Broek, 1984; Clark, Busby, Roberts, Dowell, Tong, Blamey, et al., 1987; Tong, Busby, & Clark, 1988; Skinner et al., 1992; Snik, Makhdoum, Vermeulen, Brokx, & van den Broek, 1997a; Waltzman & Cohen, 1999). These early studies confirmed predictions regarding poor outcomes with respect to open-set speech recognition. More recent reports questioning the efficacy of cochlear implantation for adults and adolescent children with prelingual deafness have yielded mixed results with some showing significant, though reduced, benefit for open-set speech understanding (Snik, Vermeulen, Geelen, Brokx, & van der Broek, 1997b; Kaplan, Shipp, Chen, Ng, & Nedzelski, 2003; Teoh, Pisoni, & Miyamoto, 2004; Klop, Briaire, Stiggelbout, & Frijns, 2007; Caposecco, Hickson, & Pedley, 2012; Firszt et al., 2012) and others with significant improvement in auditory-only speech understanding (Dowell, Dettman, Hill, Winton, Barker, & Clark, 2002). Perhaps we should have a different set of expectations for postoperative outcomes with prelingually deafened adults and older children. The focus would be centered on improved quality of life, environmental sound awareness, safety, and overall psychosocial well-being. Prelingually deafened adults have consistently reported significant improvement in subjective benefit, satisfaction, and overall communication following cochlear implantation (Zwolan, Kileny, & Telian, 1996; Klop et al., 2007; Most, Shrem, & Duvdevani, 2010; Hiraumi, Yamamoto, Sakamoto, & Ito, 2010; van Dijkhuizen, Beers, Boermans, Briaire, & Frijns, 2011; Caposecco et al., 2012); thus, it is critical to acquire preoperative subjective estimates of hearing handicap, overall quality of life, and communication effectiveness in the prelingually deafened adult implant candidate. (See Chapter 2 for guidance on the availability of self-report measures that can be used for this purpose.)

In addition to the subjective measures recommended for determining implant candidate selection for adults with prelingual hearing loss, it is important to obtain preoperative estimates of speech understanding. Although the MSTB recommends the use of CNC monosyllables, AzBio sentences, and BKB-SIN sentence recognition in noise, we might want to consider the development of a supplemental or substitution test battery when assessing pre- and post-implant performance for adults with pre- and perilingual onset of deafness. At present there are no standardized recommendations for such a modified battery. Van Dijkhuizen and colleagues (2011) recommend a new test battery for the evaluation of prelingually deafened adults to serve as both a means of determining implant candidacy and for predicting postoperative speech-perception outcomes. The primary component of this proposed battery is the inclusion of speech production intelligibility to be used as a predictive index of postoperative outcomes. Pre-implant predictions about post-implant outcomes could aid expectation management, which is a vital component in preoperative counseling.

Another consideration relative to the pre- *and* post-implant assessment of speech understanding

for prelingually deafened patients is the inclusion of easier speech metrics, particularly for the assessment of sentence recognition. The AzBio sentence corpus, as included in the MSTB recommendations, includes two male and two female talkers who speak at a normal conversational rate. The AzBio sentences have an average of seven words per sentence and are consistent with a Flesch-Kincaid grade level of 3.9 (Flesch, 1948; Kincaid, Fishburne, Rogers, & Chissom, 1975). By comparison, the HINT sentences include a single male talker who speaks at a slower rate using clear speech. The HINT sentences have an average of five words per sentence and are consistent with a Flesch-Kincaid grade level of 1.1 (Flesch, 1948; Kincaid et al., 1975). Using an easier sentence material, such as the HINT sentences (Nilsson, Soli, & Sullivan, 1994), for the assessment of speech recognition for prelingually deafened adults may be a more appropriate measurement, particularly for tracking postoperative benefit. Another suggestion would be to place more emphasis on the accuracy of phoneme recognition for monosyllabic stimuli such as CNC words. Figure 5–2 displays a hypothetical battery of tests for use with prelingually deafened adults who have limited auditory skills. As discussed in Chapters 2 and 6, more than the protocol itself, what is essential is that all clinicians in a center follow the same practice. Protocol adherence allows each implant program to generate its own normative data for patient outcomes, which significantly aids patient counseling. This also provides clinicians with the data needed to compare their clinic's outcomes to average patient performance in the literature.

Just as we must be wary of ceiling effects in our assessment metrics, we must also be aware of floor effects. If we use the metrics recommended by the MSTB for our prelingual adult recipients, we should expect to see a high proportion of these patients scoring near 0%, possibly even in the postoperative condition. Floor effects render longitudinal tracking of patient progress nearly impossible. We should not patronize our patients with the use of such simple stimuli so as to misrepresent their progress; however, we do need to utilize the most appropriate measurement tools at our disposal. As clinicians, we must be prepared to challenge our patients in assessing progress,

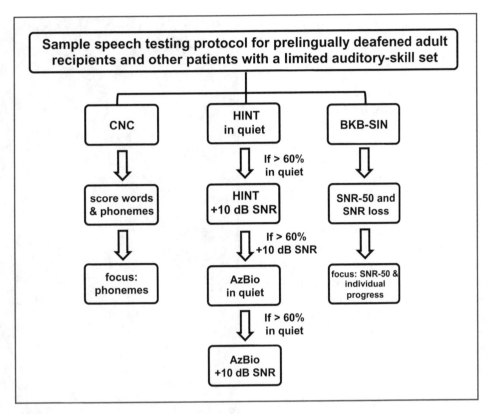

FIGURE 5–2. Sample speech-testing protocol for prelingually deafened adult recipients and other patients with a limited auditory skill set. **CNC** consonant nucleus consonant; **HINT** Hearing in Noise Test; **SNR** signal-to-noise ratio.

but also be sensitive to the fact that using metrics above the level of the patient's auditory skills will lead to frustration and discouragement. Just as we administer developmentally appropriate speech measures for our pediatric patients, the use of *auditory-skill appropriate* measures is sensible from a patient-management perspective. Should an individual center draft a testing protocol for patients with lower auditory skills, it is possible that over time the patient may demonstrate sufficient progress to a level at which the recommended MSTB can be used for assessment.

COCHLEAR IMPLANTATION FOR CHILDREN WITH SPECIAL NEEDS: GLOBAL DEVELOPMENTAL DELAY

It is well known that up to 40% of children with sensorineural hearing loss also have other medical and/or developmental comorbidities including cognitive, visual, motor, behavioral, and learning (Fortnum, Marshall & Summerfield, 2002; Gallaudet Research Institute, 2008; Roberts & Hindley, 1999; Van Naarden et al., 1999). Despite the prevalence of comorbidities in childhood hearing loss, there is currently no professional consensus regarding cochlear implantation as a viable, successful treatment option for children with special needs, particularly for those children with compromised cognition and severe global developmental delay.

An obvious, nontrivial consideration in determining cochlear implant candidacy for children with hearing loss and special needs is the difficulty in obtaining reliable behavioral estimates of hearing. In some cases, we may not be able to obtain reliable behavioral audiometric thresholds; however, given the various objective measures of auditory function we have at our disposal, confirmation of the nature and degree of hearing loss for even the nonresponsive child is possible. Furthermore, sedated magnetic resonance imaging can confirm the presence and structural status of the auditory nerve.

Expectations management is a vital component of pre-implant counseling for families. There will be those families believing that the restoration of hearing will resolve impaired cognition, behavioral issues, autism, etc. Hearing loss certainly complicates these diagnoses by restricting effective communication. Indeed, significant hearing loss confounds the interpretation of neurodevelopmental assessment, and thus it is possible to observe significant improvement in a child's behavior and overall responsiveness following cochlear implantation; however, in most cases, hearing loss is not the underlying cause of the developmental delay. This is particularly true for diagnoses including, but not limited to, agenesis of the corpus callosum, autism, cerebral palsy, Down syndrome, Fragile X syndrome, and Rett syndrome. Thus it is critical that we have the counseling skills needed to be empathetic as well as honest and realistic about what cochlear implants can and cannot do in this special population (Figure 5–3).

A recurrent theme throughout this chapter has been determining implant selection on an individual patient basis. Perhaps no other situation dictates the individuality of candidate selection and assessment more than that for children with special needs. We generally expect more modest outcomes with respect to the development of auditory skills and auditory/oral speech and language, particularly for those children exhibiting significant global developmental delay. In many reports, children with developmental delay demonstrated significant postoperative benefit in auditory perceptual skills (Waltzman, Scalchunes, & Cohen, 2000; Pyman, Blamey, Lacy, Clark, & Dowell, 2000; Hamzavi et al., 2000; Meinzen-Darr, Wiley, Grether, & Choo, 2011; Bruce, Broomfield, Henderson, Green, & Ramsden, 2011) and overall quality of life for the child and his or her family. Although our definition of what constitutes "successful outcome" will be individually tailored for each child, the presence of global developmental delay should not automatically preclude cochlear implantation.

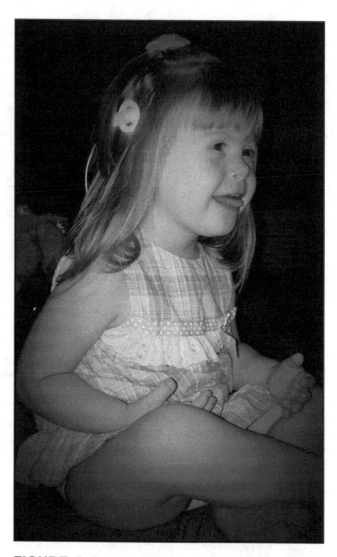

FIGURE 5–3. Savanna is an adorable 4-year-old bilateral implant recipient with Down syndrome. Savanna's mother reported that her speech, language, and overall motoric development dramatically improved following activation of her first implant at nearly 2 years of age. Savanna loves to sing and is able to do so as a result of her implants.

COCHLEAR IMPLANTATION FOR PATIENTS WITH NEUROFIBROMATOSIS TYPE 2

Neurofibromatosis type 2 (NF2) is an autosomal-dominant genetic disorder that results in the development of various nonmalignant tumors along nerves and structures within the central nervous system. Individuals with NF2 generally develop bilateral vestibular schwannomas (more commonly referred to as acoustic neuromas), which over time lead to bilateral profound deafness. Historically, aural rehabilitation for patients with NF2 has included conventional amplification until the point at which surgical removal of the tumor(s) is required. For large and invasive tumors, an auditory brainstem implant (ABI) is generally placed during neuro-otologic surgery for tumor resection. Patients with ABIs, however, typically exhibit modest postoperative speech recognition in the absence of visual cues (Colletti & Shannon, 2005; Kuchta, 2007; Goffi-Gomez et al., 2012), with many recipients never achieving open-set speech understanding.

There have been a number of reports describing successful cochlear implantation following treatment either via stereotactic radiosurgery (gamma knife) or surgical resection with neural preservation (Hoffman, Kohan, & Cohen, 1992; Tono, Ushisako, & Morimitsu, 1996; Graham, Lynch, Weber, Stollwerck, Wei, & Brookes, 1999; Temple, Axon, Ramsden, Keles, Deger, & Yucel, 1999; Ahsan, Telischi, Hodges & Balkany, 2003; Aristegui & Denia, 2005; Lustig, Yeagle, Driscoll, Blevins, Francis & Niparko, 2006; Vincenti, Pasanisi, Guida, Di Trapani, & Sanna, 2008; Tran Ba Huy, Kania, Frachet, Poncet, & Legac, 2009; Trotter & Briggs, 2010; Roehm, Mallen-St. Clair, Jethanamest, Golfinos, Shapiro, Waltzman, & Roland, 2011; Neff, Wiet, Lasak, Cohen, Pillsbury, Ramsden, & Welling 2007; Nolle, Todt, Basta, Unterberg, Mautner, & Ernst, 2003; Carlson, Breen, Driscoll, Link, Neff, Gifford & Beatty, 2012). Figure 5–4 displays individual and mean scores for the three studies that reported postoperative CNC word recognition performance for cochlear implantation with NF2. Outcomes for speech understanding can be quite variable in this population, though scores are generally much higher with a greater proportion of patients achieving open-set speech recognition than reported following ABI placement. It has been hypothesized that poorer than typical word recognition outcomes are the result of the electric signal being transmitted across a diseased neural system, which is not the case for the conventional cochlear implant recipient with cochlear hearing loss.

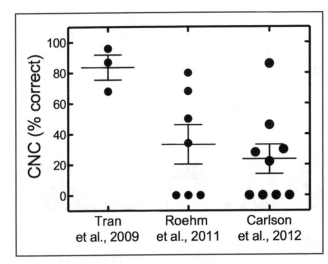

FIGURE 5–4. Postoperative CNC word recognition performance (in % correct) for three studies describing outcomes for individuals with NF2 implanted following tumor removal.

Recommendations of cochlear implantation in cases of NF2 should be accompanied with considerable patient counseling regarding outcomes and expectations. A well-known and expected scenario is that additional tumors develop along the auditory pathway; thus, it is possible that even with neural preservation following tumor resection, disease progression may ultimately restrict or completely terminate reliable function of the implant.

CONCLUSION

Candidacy criteria have dramatically evolved over the past several decades, and cochlear implants are no longer only for individuals with profound sensorineural deafness. A number of studies have demonstrated the efficacy of cochlear implants for individuals falling outside current candidacy indications with respect to audiometric thresholds (severity, configuration, and symmetry), speech understanding, age, etiology, and developmental abilities. As stressed throughout Chapters 2 and 3, it is of critical importance that implant candidate selection be determined on an individual basis considering the whole patient—rather than focusing entirely on the audiogram. Although indications are in place to provide guidance for clinicians and patients, there will never be a substitute for the professional clinical judgment of the interdisciplinary cochlear implant team.

REFERENCES

Adunka, O., Buss, E., Clark, M., Pillsbury, H. C., & Buchman, C. A. (2008). Effect of preoperative residual hearing on speech perception after cochlear implantation. *Laryngoscope, 118,* 2044–2049.

Ahsan, S., Telischi, F., Hodges, A., & Balkany, T. (2003). Cochlear implantation concurrent with translabyrinthine acoustic neuroma resection. *Laryngoscope, 113,* 472–474.

Amoodi, H. A., Mick, P. T., Shipp, D. B., Friesen, L. M., Nedzelski, J. M., Chen, J. M., et al. (2011). The effects of unilateral cochlear implantation on the tinnitus handicap inventory and the influence on quality of life. *Laryngoscope, 121*(7), 1536–1540.

Aristegui, M., & Denia, A. (2005). Simultaneous cochlear implantation and translabyrinthine removal of vestibular schwannoma in an only hearing ear: Report of two cases (neurofibromatosis type 2 and unilateral vestibular schwannoma). *Otology & Neurotology, 26,* 205–210.

Arndt, S., Aschendorff, A., Laszig, R., Beck, R., Schild, C., Kroeger, S., Ihorst, G., & Wesarg, T. (2011). Comparison of pseudobinaural hearing to real binaural hearing rehabilitation after cochlear implantation in patients with unilateral deafness and tinnitus. *Otology & Neurotology, 32,* 39–47.

Beijen, J. W., Mylanus, E. A., Leeuw, A. R., & Snik, A. F. (2008). Should a hearing aid in the contralateral ear be recommended for children with a unilateral cochlear implant? *Annals of Otology, Rhinology and Laryngology, 117*(6), 397–403.

Bergeson, T. R., Houston, D. M., & Miyamoto, R. T. (2010). Effects of congenital hearing loss and cochlear implantation on audiovisual speech perception in infants and children. *Restorative Neurology and Neuroscience, 28,* 157–165.

Bradham T., & Jones, G. (2008). Cochlear implant candidacy in the United States: prevalence in children 12 months to 6 years of age. *International Journal of Pediatric Otorhinolaryngology, 72,* 1023–1028.

Bruce, I. A., Broomfield, S. J., Henderson, L., Green, K. M., & Ramsden, R. T. (2011). Cochlear implantation in Donnai-Barrow syndrome. *Cochlear Implants International, 12*(1), 60–63.

Buechner, A., Brendel, M., Lesinski-Schiedat, A., Wenzel, G., Frohne-Buechner, C., Jaeger, B., et al. (2010). Cochlear implantation in unilateral deaf subjects associated with ipsilateral tinnitus. *Otology & Neurotology, 31*(9), 1381–1385.

Caposecco, A., Hickson, L., & Pedley, K. (2012). Cochlear implant outcomes in adults and adolescents with early-onset hearing loss. *Ear and Hearing, 33*(2), 209–220.

Carlson, M.C., Breen, J.T., Driscoll, C. L. W., Link, M. J., Neff, B. A., Gifford, R. H., & Beatty, C. W. (2012). Cochlear implantation in patients with neurofibromatosis type 2: variables affecting auditory performance. *Otology & Neurotology, 33,* 853–862.

Ching, T. Y., Hill, M., Brew, J., Incerti, P., Priolo, S., Rushbrook, E., et al. (2005). The effect of auditory experience on speech perception, localization, and functional performance of children who use a cochlear implant and a hearing aid in opposite ears. *International Journal of Audiology, 44*(12), 677–690.

Ching, T. Y., Incerti, P., Hill, M., & van Wanrooy, E. (2006). An overview of binaural advantages for children and adults who use binaural/bimodal hearing devices. *Audiology and Neurotology, 11*(Suppl 1), 6–11.

Ching, T. Y., Psarros, C., Hill, M., Dillon, H., & Incerti, P. (2001). Should children who use cochlear implants wear hearing aids in the opposite ear? *Ear and Hearing, 22,* 365–380.

Ching, T. Y., van Wanrooy, E., & Dillon, H. (2007). Binaural-bimodal fitting or bilateral implantation for managing severe to profound deafness: A review. *Trends in Amplification, 11,* 161–192

Clark, G. M., Busby, P. A. , Roberts, S. A.,Dowell, R. C., Tong, Y. C., Blamey, et al. (1987). Preliminary results for the cochlear corporation multielectrode intracochlear implant in six prelingually deaf patients. *American Journal of Otology, 8,* 234–239.

Cohen, R. A., & Martines, M. E. (2012). Health insurance coverage: Early release of estimates from the national health interview survey, 2011. National Center for Health Statistics. June 2012. Available at: http://www.cdc.gov/nchs/nhis/releases.htm

Colletti, V., Carner, M., Miorelli, V., Guida, M., Colletti, L., & Fiorino, F. G. (2005). Cochlear implantation at under 12 months: Report on 10 patients. *Laryngoscope, 115,* 445–449.

Colletti, V., & Shannon, R. V. (2005). Open set speech perception with auditory brainstem implant? *Laryngoscope, 115*(11), 1974–1978.

Cosetti, M., & Roland, J. T. (2010). Cochlear implantation in the very young child: issues unique to the under-1 population. *Trends in Amplification, 14,* 46–57.

Cowan, R. S., Deldot, J., Barker, E. J., Sarant, J. Z., Pegg, P., Dettman, S., et al. (1997). Speech perception results for children with implants with different levels of preoperative residual hearing. *American Journal of Otology, 18*(Suppl 6), S125–S126.

Dettman, S. J., D'Costa, W. A., Dowell, R. C., Winton, E. J., Hill, K. L., & Williams, S. S. (2004). Cochlear implants for children with significant residual hearing. *Archives of Otolaryngology Head and Neck Surgery, 130,* 612–618.

Dettman, S. J., Pinder, D., Briggs, R. J., Dowell, R. C., & Leigh, J. R. (2007). Communication development in children who receive the cochlear implant younger than 12 months: Risks versus benefits. *Ear and Hearing, 28,* 11S–18S.

Dowell, R. C., Dettman, S. J., Hill, K., Winton, E., Barker, E. J., & Clark, G. M. (2002). Speech perception outcomes in older children who use multichannel cochlear implants: Older is not always poorer. *Annals of Otology, Rhinology and Laryngology Supplment, 189,* 97–101.

Eisenberg, L. S., Martinez, A. S., Holowecky, S. R., & Pogorelsky, S. (2002). Recognition of lexically controlled words and sentences by children with normal hearing and children with cochlear implants. *Ear and Hearing, 23,* 450–462.

El Fata, F., James, C. J., Laborde, M. L., & Fraysse, B. (2009). How much residual hearing is "useful" for music perception with cochlear implants? *Audiology and Neuro-Otology, 1,* 14–21.

Firszt, J. B., Holden, L. K., Reeder, R. M., Cowdrey, L., & King, S. (2012). Cochlear implantation in adults with asymmetric hearing loss. *Ear and Hearing, 33*(4), 521–533.

Flesch, R. (1948). A new readability yardstick. *Journal of Applied Psychology, 32,* 221–233.

Fortnum, H. M., Marshall, D. H., & Summerfield, A. Q. (2002). Epidemiology of the UK population of hearing-impaired children, including characteristics of those with and without cochlear implants—audiology, aetiology, comorbidity and affluence. *International Journal of Audiology, 4,* 170–179.

Gallaudet Research Institute (2008). Regional and National Summary Report of Data from the 2007–08 Annual Survey of Deaf and Hard of Hearing Children and Youth. Washington, DC: GRI, Gallaudet University.

Gantz, B. J., Rubinstein, J. T., Tyler, R. S., Teagle, H. F., Cohen, N. L., Waltzman, et al. (2000). Long-term results of cochlear implants in children with residual hearing. *Annals of Otology, Rhinology and Laryngology Supplement, 185,* 33–36.

G090032/S005. (2011). *Evaluation of revised indication for determining adult cochlear implant candidacy, investigational device exemption.* Cochlear Americas, Centennial, CO.

Gifford, R. H., Dorman, M. F., McKarns, S. A., & Spahr, A. J. (2007). Combined electric and contralateral acoustic hearing: Word and sentence recognition with bimodal hearing. *Journal of Speech Language and Hearing Research, 50,* 835–843.

Gifford, R. H., Dorman, M. F., Shallop, J. K., & Sydlowski, S. A. (2010). Evidence for the expansion of adult cochlear implant candidacy. *Ear and Hearing, 31,* 186–194.

Gifford, R. H., Shallop, J. K., & Peterson, A. M. (2008). Speech recognition materials and ceiling effects: considerations for cochlear implant programs. *Audiology & Neurotology, 13,* 193–205.

Goffi-Gomez, M. V., Magalhães, A. T., Brito Neto, R., Tsuji, R. K., Gomes Mde, Q., & Bento, R. F. (2012). Auditory brainstem implant outcomes and MAP parameters: Report of experiences in adults and children. *International Journal of Pediatric Otorhinolaryngology, 76*(2), 257–264.

Graham, J., Lynch, C., Weber, B., Stollwerck, L., Wei, J., & Brookes, G. (1999). The magnetless Clarion cochlear implant in a patient with neurofibromatosis 2. *Journal of Laryngology & Otology, 113,* 458–463.

Habib, M. G. , Waltzman, S. B., Tajudeen, B., & Svirsky, M. A. (2010). Speech production intelligibility of early implanted pediatric cochlear implant users. *International Journal of Pediatric Otorhinolaryngology, 74,* 855–859.

Hamzavi, J., Baumgartner, W. D., Egelierler, B., Franz, P., Schenk, B., & Gstoettner, W. (2000). Follow up of cochlear implanted handicapped children. *International Journal of Pediatric Otorhinolaryngology, 56,* 169–174.

Hayes,H,. Geers, A. E., Treiman, R., & Moog, J. S. (2009). Receptive vocabulary development in deaf children with cochlear implants: achievement in an intensive auditory-oral educational setting. *Ear and Hearing, 30,* 128–135.

Hinderink, J. B., Snik, A. F., Mens, L. H., Brokx, J. P., & Van den Broek, P. (1984). Performance of prelingually or postlingually deafened adults who were using a single or multichannel cochlear implant. *Ear, Nose & Throat Journal, 73*(3), 180–183.

Hiraumi, H., Yamamoto, N., Sakamoto, T., & Ito J. (2010). Cochlear implantation in patients with prelingual hearing loss. *Acta Otolaryngologica Supplement, 563,* 4–10.

Hoffman, R. A., Kohan, D., & Cohen, N. L. (1992). Cochlear implants in the management of bilateral acoustic neuromas. *American Journal of Otology, 13*, 525–528.

Holt, R. F., Kirk, K. I., Eisenberg, L. S., Martinez, A. S., & Campbell, W. (2005). Spoken word recognition development in children with residual hearing using cochlear implants and hearing aids in opposite ears. *Ear and Hearing, 26*(4 Suppl), 82S–91S.

Houston, D. M., & Miyamoto, R. T. (2010). Effects of early auditory experience on word learning and speech perception in deaf children with cochlear implants: Implications for sensitive periods of language development. *Otology and Neurotology, 31*(8), 1248–1253.

Houston, D. M., Stewart, J., Moberly, A., Hollich, G., & Miyamoto, R. T. (2012). Word learning in deaf children with cochlear implants: Effects of early auditory experience. *Developmental Science, 15*, 448–461.

Huart, S., & Sammeth, C. (2009). Identifying cochlear implant candidates in the hearing aid dispensing practice. *Hearing Review, 16*(5), 24–32.

James, A. L., & Papsin, B. C. (2004). Cochlear implant surgery at 12 months of age or younger. *Laryngoscope, 114*, 2191–2195.

Kaplan, D. M., Shipp, D. B., Chen, J. M., Ng, A. H., & Nedzelski, J. M. (2003). Early-deafened adult cochlear implant users: Assessment of outcomes. *Journal of Otolaryngology, 32*(4), 245–249.

Kincaid, J. P., Fishburne, R. P., Rogers, R. L., & Chissom, B. S. (1975). Derivation of new readability formulas (Automated Readability Index, Fog Count and Flesch Reading Ease Formula) for Navy enlisted personnel. *Research Branch Report 8–75*. Millington, TN: Naval Technical Training, U.S. Naval Air Station, Memphis, TN.

Kleinjung, T., Steffens, T., Strutz, J., & Langguth, B. (2009). Curing tinnitus with a cochlear implant in a patient with unilateral sudden deafness: A case report. *Cases Journal, 18*(2), 7462.

Klop, W. M., Briaire, J. J., Stiggelbout, A. M., & Frijns, J. H. (2007). Cochlear implant outcomes and quality of life in adults with prelingual deafness. *Laryngoscope, 117*(11), 1982–1987.

Kochkin, S., Beck, D. L., Christensen, L. A., Compton-Conley, C., Fligor, B. J., Kricos, P. B., et al. (2010). MarkeTrak VIII: The impact of the hearing healthcare professional on hearing aid user success. *Hearing Review, 17*, 12–34.

Kuchta, J. (2007). Twenty-five years of auditory brainstem implants: Perspectives. *Acta Neurochirurgica Supplement, 97*(Pt 2), 443–449.

Leigh, J., Dettman, S., Dowell, R. C., & Sarant, J. (2011). Evidence-based approach for making cochlear implant recommendations for infants with residual hearing. *Ear and Hearing, 32*, 313–322.

Liu, H., Zhang, H., Bentler, R. A., Mo, L., Han, D., & Zhang, L. (2011). Audiometric records analysis in a clinical population in China. *ORL Journal for Otorhinolaryngology and Its Related Specialties, 73*(5), 237–245.

Lustig, L. R., Yeagle, J., Driscoll, C. L., Blevins, N., Francis, H., & Niparko, J. K. (2006). Cochlear implantation in patients with neurofibromatosis type 2 and bilateral vestibular schwannoma. *Otology & Neurotology, 27*, 512–518.

Margolis, R. H., & Saly, G. L. (2008). Asymmetric hearing loss: Definition, validation, and prevalence. *Otology & Neurotology, 29*(4), 422–431.

Mehra, S., Eavey, R. D., & Keamy, D. G. Jr. (2009). The epidemiology of hearing impairment in the United States. *Otolaryngology — Head and Neck Surgery, 140*(4), 461–472.

Meinzen-Derr, J., Wiley, S., Grether, S., & Choo, D. I. (2011). Children with cochlear implants and developmental disabilities: A language skills study with developmentally matched hearing peers. *Research in Developmental Disabilities, 32*, 757–767.

Miyamoto, R. T., Hay-McCutcheon, M. J., Kirk, K. I., Houston, D. M., & Bergeson-Dana, T. (2008). Language skills of profoundly deaf children who received cochlear implants under 12 months of age: A preliminary study. *Acta Oto-Laryngologica, 128*, 373–377.

Miyamoto, R. T., Houston, D. M., & Bergeson, T. (2005). Cochlear implantation in deaf infants. *Laryngoscope, 115*, 1376–1380.

Mok, M., Galvin, K. L., Dowell, R. C., & McKay, C. M. (2010). Speech perception benefit for children with a cochlear implant and a hearing aid in opposite ears and children with bilateral cochlear implants. *Audiology and Neurotology, 15*(1), 44–56.

Mok, M., Grayden, D., Dowell, R. C., & Lawrence, D. (2006). Speech perception for adults who use hearing aids in conjunction with cochlear implants in opposite ears. *Journal of Speech, Language, and Hearing Research, 49*, 338–351.

Mondaine, M., Sillon, M., Vieu, A., Levi, A., Reuilard-Artieres, F., & Deguine, O. (2002). Cochlear implantation in prelingually deafened children with residual hearing. *International Journal of Pediatric Otorhinolaryngology, 63*, 91–97.

Moog, J. S., & Geers, A. E. (2010). Early educational placement and later language outcomes for children with cochlear implants. *Otology & Neurotology, 31*, 1315–1319.

Most, T., Shrem, H., & Duvdevani, I. (2010). Cochlear implantation in late-implanted adults with prelingual deafness. *American Journal of Otolaryngology, 31*(6), 418–423.

Neff, B. A., Wiet, R. M., Lasak, J. M., Cohen, N. L., Pillsbury, H.C., Ramsden, R. T., & Welling, D. B. (2007). Cochlear implantation in the neurofibromatosis type 2 patient: Long-term follow-up. *Laryngoscope, 117,* 1069–1072.

NIH. (2011). Cochlear implants. NIH publication no. 11-4798. Content updated March 2011. Retrieved May 18, 2012, from http://www.nidcd.nih.gov/health/hearing/pages/coch.aspx

Nilsson, M., Soli, S., & Sullivan, J. (1994). Development of the Hearing in Noise test for the measurement of speech reception thresholds in quiet and in noise. *Journal of the Acoustical Society of America, 95,* 1085–1099.

Niparko, J. K., Tobey, E. A., Thal, D. J., Eisenberg, L. S., Wang, N. Y., Quittner, A. L., et al. (2010). Spoken language development in children following cochlear implantation. *Journal of the American Medical Association, 303,* 1498–1506.

Nolle, C., Todt, I., Basta, D., Unterberg, A., Mautner, V. F., & Ernst, A. (2003). Cochlear implantation after acoustic tumour resection in neurofibromatosis type 2: Impact of intra- and postoperative neural response telemetry monitoring. *ORL Journal for Otorhinolaryngology and Its Relatated Specialties, 65,* 230–234.

Punte, A. K., Vermeire, K., Hofkens, A., De Bodt, M., De Ridder, D., & van de Heyning, P. (2011). Cochlear implantation as a durable tinnitus treatment in single-sided deafness. *Cochlear Implants International, 12*(Suppl 1), S26–S29.

Pyman, B., Blamey, P., Lacy, P., Clark, G., & Dowell, R. (2000). The development of speech perception in children using cochlear implants: Effects of etiologic factors and delayed milestones. *American Journal of Otology, 21,* 57–61.

Ramos, Á., Polo, R., Masgoret, E., Artiles, O., Lisner, I., Zaballos, M. L., et al. (2012). Cochlear implant in patients with sudden unilateral sensorineural hearing loss and associated tinnitus. *Acta Otorrinolaringológica Española, 63*(1), 15–20.

Roberts, C., & Hindley, P. (1999). The assessment and treatment of deaf children with psychiatric disorders. *Journal of Child Psychology and Psychiatry, 40,* 151–167.

Roehm, P. C., Mallen-St. Clair, J., Jethanamest, D., Golfinos, J. G., Shapiro, W., Waltzman, S., & Roland, R.T. (2011). Auditory rehabilitation of patients with neurofibromatosis type 2 by using cochlear implants. *Journal of Neurosurgery, 115,* 827–834.

Skinner, M. W., Binzer, S. M., Fears, B. T., Holden, T. A., Jenison, V. W., & Nettles, E. J. (1992). Study of the performance of four prelinguistically or perilinguistically deaf patients with a multi-electrode, intracochlear implant. *Laryngoscope, 102,* 797–806.

Snik, A. F., Makhdoum, M. J., Vermeulen, A. M., Brokx, J. P., & van den Broek, P. (1997a). The relation between age at the time of cochlear implantation and long-term speech perception abilities in congenitally deaf subjects. *International Journal of Pediatric Otorhinolaryngology, 20*(4), 121–131.

Snik, A. F., Vermeulen, A. M., Geelen, C. P., Brokx, J. P., & van der Broek, P. (1997b). Speech perception performance of congenitally deaf patients with a cochlear implant: the effect of age at implantation. *American Journal of Otology, 18*(6 Suppl), S138–S139.

Stern, R. E., Yueh, B., Lewis, C., Norton, S., & Sie, K. C. (2005). Recent epidemiology of pediatric cochlear implantation in the United States: Disparity among children of different ethnicity and socioeconomic status. *Laryngoscope, 115*(1), 125–131

Straatman, L. V., Rietveld, A. C., Beijen, J., Mylanus, E. A., & Mens, L. H. (2010). Advantage of bimodal fitting in prosody perception for children using a cochlear implant and a hearing aid. *Journal of the Acoustical Society of America, 128*(4), 1884–1895.

Sucher, C. M., & McDermott, H. J. (2009). Bimodal stimulation: benefits for music perception and sound quality. *Cochlear Implants International, 1,* 96–99.

Tajudeen, B. A., Waltzman, S. B., Jethanamest, D., & Svirsky, M. A. (2010). Speech perception in congenitally deaf children receiving cochlear implants in the first year of life. *Otology & Neurotology, 31,*1254–1260.

Temple, R. H., Axon, P. R., Ramsden, R. T., Keles, N., Deger, K., & Yucel, E. (1999). Auditory rehabilitation in neurofibromatosis type 2: A case for cochlear implantation. *Journal of Laryngology & Otology, 113,* 161–163.

Teoh, S. W., Pisoni, D. B., & Miyamoto, R. T. (2004). Cochlear implantation in adults with prelingual deafness. Part I. Clinical results. *Laryngoscope, 114,* 1536–1540.

Tomblin, J. B., Barker, B. A., Spencer, L. J., Zhang, X., & Gantz, B. J. (2005). The effect of age at cochlear implant initial stimulation on expressive language growth in infants and toddlers. *Journal of Speech Language and Hearing Research, 48,* 853–867.

Tomblin, J. B., Spencer, L., Flock, S., Tyler, R., & Gantz, B. (1999). A comparison of language achievement in children with cochlear implants and children using hearing aids. *Journal of Speech and Language, 42,* 497–509.

Tong, Y. C., Busby, P. A., & Clark, G. M. (1988). Perceptual studies on cochlear implant patients with early onset of profound hearing impairment prior to normal development of auditory, speech, and language skills. *Journal of the Acoustical Society of America, 84*(3), 951–962.

Tono, T., Ushisako, Y., & Morimitsu, T. (1996). Cochlear implantation in an intralabyrinthine acoustic neuroma patient after resection of an intracanalicular tumour. *Journal of Laryngology and Otology, 110,* 570–573.

Tran Ba Huy, P., Kania, R., Frachet, B., Poncet, C., & Legac, M. S. (2009). Auditory rehabilitation with cochlear implantation in patients with neurofibromatosis type 2. *Acta Otolaryngologica, 129,* 971–975.

Tremblay, G., Bergeron, F., & Ferron, P. (2008). Over-the-fence cochlear implantation: Is it worthwhile? *Journal of Otolaryngology—Head and Neck Surgery, 37*(3), 440–445.

Trotter, M. I., & Briggs, R. J. (2010). Cochlear implantation in neurofibromatosis type 2 after radiation therapy. *Otology & Neurotology, 31,* 216–219.

Tyler, R. S., Parkinson, A. J., Wilson, B. S., Witt, S., Preece, J. P., & Noble, W. (2002). Patients utilizing a hearing aid and a cochlear implant: speech perception and localization. *Ear and Hearing, 23,* 98–105.

Valencia, D. M., Rimell, F. L., Friedman, B. J., Oblander, M. R., & Helmbrecht, J. (2008). Cochlear implantation in infants less than 12 months of age. *International Journal of Pediatric Otorhinolaryngology, 72,* 767–773.

van de Heyning, P., Vermeire, K., Diebl, M., Nopp, P., Anderson, I., & De Ridder, D. (2008). Incapacitating unilateral tinnitus in single-sided deafness treated by cochlear implantation. *Annals of Otology, Rhinology and Laryngology, 117*(9), 645–652.

van Dijkhuizen, J. N., Beers, M., Boermans, P. P., Briaire, J. J., & Frijns, J. H. (2011). Speech intelligibility as a predictor of cochlear implant outcome in prelingually deafened adults. *Ear and Hearing, 32*(4), 445–458.

Van Naarden, K., Decoufle, P., & Caldwell, K. (1999). Prevalence and characteristics of children with serious hearing impairment in metropolitan Atlanta, 1991–1993. *Pediatrics, 103,* 570–575.

Vermeire, K., & van de Heyning, P. (2009). Binaural hearing after cochlear implantation in subjects with unilateral sensorineural deafness and tinnitus. *Audiology and Neurotology, 14*(3), 163–171.

Vincenti, V., Pasanisi, E., Guida, M., Di Trapani, G., & Sanna, M. (2008). Hearing rehabilitation in neurofibromatosis type 2 patients: Cochlear versus auditory brainstem implantation. *Audiology and Neurotology, 13,* 273–280.

Waltzman, S. B., & Cohen, N. L. (1999). Implantation of patients with prelingual long-term deafness. *Annals of Otology, Rhinology and Laryngology, 108,* 84–87.

Waltzman, S. B., & Roland, J. T., Jr. (2005). Cochlear implantation in children younger than 12 months. *Pediatrics, 116,* 487–493.

Waltzman, S. B., Scalchunes, V., & Cohen, N. L. (2000). Performance of multiply handicapped children using cochlear implants. *American Journal of Otology, 21,* 329–335.

Wilson, B., & Dorman, M. (2008). Interfacing Sensors with the nervous system: Lessons from the development and success of the cochlear implant. *IEEE Sensors Journal, 8,* 131–147.

Winton, L., Hollow, R., & Dettman, S. J (2002). Cochlear implant speech perception selection criteria: Who is a candidate now? In *Proceedings of the XXVI International Congress of Audiology,* March 17–21, Melbourne, Australia.

Wu, E., Zardouz, S., Rothholtz, V., German, M., & Djalilian, H. (2010). Primary care physicians' knowledge of cochlear implantation. *Otolaryngology—Head and Neck Surgery, 143,* P244.

Yoshinago-Itano, C., Baca, R. L., & Sedey, A. L. (2010). Describing the trajectory of language development in the presence of severe-to-profound hearing loss: A closer look at children with cochlear implants versus hearing aids. *Otology & Neurotology, 31,* 1268–1274.

Zwolan, T. A., Kileny, P. R., & Telian, S. A. (1996). Self-report of cochlear implant use and satisfaction by prelingually deafened adults. *Ear and Hearing, 17*(3), 198–210.

6

Elements of Postoperative Assessment: Adult Implant Recipients

René H. Gifford

INTRODUCTION

Determining a reliable and efficacious assessment protocol for the evaluation of speech perception has been, and will continue to be, an evolutionary process. Mackersie (2002) describes the ideal speech perception test as being reliable, highly sensitive to differences between testing conditions, and having a high degree of correlation with real-world speech understanding. Another factor, across-test correlation or agreement, is also an important consideration in the choice of metrics. As discussed in Chapter 2, the Minimum Speech Test Battery (MSTB) represents current best practices for pre- and post-implant assessment of speech recognition for adult implant candidates and recipients. There are, however, many factors to be considered in the postoperative assessment of adult implant recipients other than the *exact measures* to be used.

This chapter discusses the process of postoperative assessment of performance for adult cochlear implant recipients of including aspects to be considered from the perspective of all members of the implant team.

POST-IMPLANT AUDIOLOGIC EVALUATION

Assessment of Acoustic Hearing Status

Implanted Ear

As mentioned in Chapter 2, preoperative assessments include obtaining audiometric thresholds for octave frequencies 125 to 8000 Hz. Thresholds at 125 Hz are particularly important given that otologists, audiologists, and even patients are increasingly aware of the possibilities of hearing preservation with cochlear implantation (e.g., Gstoettner et al., 2008; Gantz et al., 2009; Carlson et al., 2011; Skarzynski, Lorens, Piotrowska, & Anderson, 2006). It is recommended that postoperative audiometric testing be completed first at the initial activation appointment. This test point provides us with the clearest picture of the impact that the surgical placement of the device has had on residual cochlear function. It also provides a baseline against which future measurements of residual acoustic hearing can be compared.

At this initial activation appointment, obtaining both air-conduction and bone-conduction thresholds is critical. The reason is that residual blood and/or fluid may still be present, from the surgical procedure, in the middle ear space. Tympanograms can also be completed and can verify the presence of fluid, though it is recommended that the audiology team first discuss this protocol with the surgical team to gain medical clearance, particularly for initial activations occurring sooner than 2 weeks after surgery.

In cases of hearing preservation, it is our role as clinicians to monitor this hearing over time. Over the first year of implant use, obtaining pure-tone thresholds in the implanted ear *at least one other time* beyond the initial activation appointment is recommended. This is particularly true in cases for which a conductive overlay was initially present. It is the responsibility of each program to develop its own protocols regarding postoperative hearing assessment in the implanted ear. It makes practical sense to assess hearing in the implanted ear at intervals that also include sound booth testing, such as the 6- and/or 12-month appointments. The assessment of residual hearing in the implanted ear will be an issue of further audiologic management as we investigate the possibility of providing acoustic amplification in that ear.

Nonimplanted Ear (Bimodal Listeners)

In addition to assessing residual hearing in the implanted ear, we must also continue to manage the hearing and associated effectiveness and appropriateness of amplification in the nonimplanted ear for our bimodal patients. All too often cochlear implant audiologists focus so much on the implanted ear that the nonimplanted ear goes unnoticed. We must not forget that in order to assess postoperative speech recognition in the best-aided condition, we should complete regular pure tone audiometric testing *and* probe-microphone measurements of the hearing aid to verify settings. According to the American Academy of Audiology's Guidelines for the Audiologic Management of Adult Hearing Impairment (Valente et al., 2006), electroacoustic verification of hearing aid settings should be completed, at a minimum, on an annual basis. Hearing aid verification, however, is only as good as the accuracy of one's audiometric thresholds; thus, we should also be assessing hearing in the nonimplanted ear on an annual basis.

Cochlear Implant "Aided" Audiometric Thresholds

Hearing aid audibility can be measured via SPL in the ear canal at various input signal levels. Cochlear implants, however, transmit the signal across the skin via radio-frequency transmission; thus, a physical output level cannot be *directly* measured. This does not mean that we cannot attempt to estimate minimum audibility for a recipient's program. Skinner and colleagues (1997, 1999) discussed the function of sound field audiometric thresholds for determining the minimum audibility available for implant recipients. On the basis of their work, it has become standard practice to optimize cochlear implant mapping to achieve aided sound field thresholds in the range of 20 to 30 dB HL (for 250 to 6000 Hz) for adult recipients. Documenting sound field thresholds in the range of 20 to 30 dB HL provides us with an assurance of audibility for low-level stimuli, such as "soft" speech (e.g., Skinner et al., 1997).

Given that we will already be in the sound booth obtaining aided sound field thresholds for the implanted ear, clinicians might be tempted to substitute functional gain measures for probe-microphone measurements (for bimodal listeners). This should be avoided, because functional gain measures do not verify hearing aid settings, do not provide information regarding the input/output characteristics of hearing aids and thus cannot verify ear canal audibility for multiple input levels in the range of low-, high-, and conversational-level speech. In 2006, the American Academy of Audiology published the *Guidelines for the Audiologic Management of Adult Hearing Impairment* (Valente et al., 2006), which states "prescribed gain from a validated prescriptive method should be verified using a probe microphone approach that is referenced to ear canal SPL." Thus, functional gain measures are *not* appropriate for verification of hearing aid settings as part of the postoperative assessment.

Microphone Check

Another important note is that although aided sound field thresholds provide verification of implant mapping for low-level inputs, there is no substitution for an old-fashioned mic check. Pediatric audiologists routinely listen to implant processor microphones to check for low-level humming, static, or any variation of compromised sound quality. One might argue that mic checks are even more important for adult implant recipients because most pediatric recipients have parents, educators, and clinicians who routinely check for microphone issues. This is yet another tool for postoperative assessment of performance.

Calibration and Test Conditions

Sound field calibration is completely dependent on the test conditions for the patients in the test booth. For adult sound field audiometry, the loudspeaker is typically placed directly in front of the listener (0° azimuth) at a distance of approximately 1 to 1.5 m (approximately 3.3 to 4.9 feet); thus, if a sound booth is being used exclusively for adult hearing assessment, the sound field will most likely be calibrated for loudspeaker placement at 0° azimuth. In many audiology clinics, however, sound booths are set up such that both adults and children can be tested, that is, there are loudspeakers placed at ±45 to 90° allowing for visual reinforcement audiometry. If this is the case, the sound field will most likely be calibrated assuming loudspeaker placement to the side of the listener (at either ±45 to 90°); thus, it is important that the appropriate correction factors be used when placing an adult listener in the booth facing the loudspeaker. Table 6–1 displays the frequency specific correction factors to be used when characterizing sound-field audiometric thresholds in a room that was cali-

Table 6–1. Frequency-Specific Correction Factors for Sound-Field Threshold Estimation Referencing Calibration at 0° Azimuth

Frequency (Hz)	45° (dB)	90° (dB)
125	0.5	1.0
250	1.0	2.0
500	3.0	4.5
750	3.5	3.0
1000	4.0	5.5
1500	1.5	0.0
2000	3.0	2.0
3000	5.0	2.5
4000	4.0	−0.5
6000	7.5	9.5
8000	5.5	8.5

brated for 0° azimuth (ANSI S3.21-2004; ISO 8253-2, 1998). If you are unsure whether your audiometer sound field has been calibrated for 0°, 45°, or 90° azimuth, consult your audiometer calibration certificate or acoustical engineer responsible for calibration.

Stimulus for Testing: Frequency-Modulated Tones and Narrow-Band Noise

There are just two types of audiometer-derived stimuli appropriate for obtaining sound field thresholds: frequency-modulated (FM) or warbled tones and narrow-band noise. All audiologists should be aware of the need for FM or warbled tones in the sound field to avoid problems associated with standing waves; however, many clinicians may not be aware of issues surrounding the use of narrow-band noise for sound-field threshold estimation. All audiometers are calibrated for narrow-band noise presentation via headphones or insert earphones, for effective masking levels. Not all audiometers, however, are calibrated for narrow-band noise presentation via loudspeaker. Newer computer-based audiometers come equipped with a narrower band noise stimulus that is calibrated for sound-field audiometry and has steeper filter slopes. The steeper filter slopes allow for more accurate, frequency specific threshold estimation than using narrow-band noise, which is intended for masking purposes.

SPEECH-RECOGNITION TESTING

Speech-Perception Metrics

As discussed in Chapter 2, much of the preoperative assessment in this section can also be found in the MSTB manual, which was revised in 2011 and can be downloaded for free at http://www.auditorypotential.com/MSTB.html.

The most important aspect surrounding the administration of speech recognition metrics as recommended by the MSTB involves the use of recorded speech materials. As shown in Chapter 2, Figures 2–1A and 2–1B, word-recognition scores obtained via monitored live voice (MLV) and with recorded stimuli can vary by as much as 80 percentage points for a single listener; thus, *use of MLV for the assessment of speech recognition for adult implant recipients is not valid practice.* Some clinicians argue that poorer-performing recipients, such as prelingually deafened adults, require the use of MLV for assessing speech recognition; however, as discussed in Chapter 5, we may want to consider the development of a supplemental or substitution test battery when assessing pre- and post-implant performance for adults with pre- and perilingual onset of deafness. As we have been cognizant of ceiling effects with previously used metrics of speech recognition for implant recipients, such as the Central Institute for the Deaf (CID; Silverman & Hirsh, 1955) sentences, City University of New York (CUNY) sentences, and Hearing in Noise Test (HINT; Nilsson, Soli, & Sullivan, 1994) sentences, we must also be wary of floor effects. Figure 5–2 as displayed in Chapter 5 provides an example of a hypothetical battery of tests for use with prelingually deafened adults

who have limited auditory skills. More than the protocol itself, what is essential is that all clinicians in a center follow the same practice with recorded stimuli. Protocol adherence allows each implant program to generate its own normative data for patient outcomes, which significantly aids patient counseling. This also provides clinics with the data needed to compare outcomes with those of average patient performance as reported in the literature. Furthermore, because most implant programs have multiple clinicians, adherence to protocol along with the use of recorded stimuli allows for clinician substitution without sacrificing assessment accuracy. Although we may use a specialized battery of tests for poorer performing patients, it is important to recognize that over time, a patient may demonstrate sufficient progress to a level at which the recommended MSTB may be used.

Table 6–2 displays the audiometric and speech recognition protocol as outlined in the MSTB for adult implant recipients. The recommended test battery has been estimated at approximately 30 to 45 min per listening condition. The recommended battery includes postoperative assessment of (1) unaided audiometric thresholds in the implanted ear; (2) aided sound field thresholds for the implanted ear(s); (3) speech recognition performance using CNC words (Peterson & Lehiste, 1962), AzBio sentences (Spahr et al., 2012), and AzBio sentences presented in multitalker babble using a +5 dB signal-to-noise ratio or one list pair of the Bamford-Kowal-Bench-Sentence-in-noise (BKB-SIN) test (Killion, Niquette, Revit, & Skinner, 2001; Etymotic Research, 2005); and (4) administration of questionnaires assessing perceived benefit and/or quality of life.

Testing Conditions

The testing conditions for assessing postoperative performance are not widely agreed upon among clinicians. The MSTB manual does not provide a recommendation regarding the listening conditions or the frequency of testing for implant recipients. In 2009, a working group of clinicians, scientists, and manufacturer representatives published a recommended postoperative testing

Table 6–2. Test Battery for Postoperative Assessment of Outcomes in Adults

		Maximum time (min)
Hearing assessment in implanted ear(s)		
Pure-tone audiometry-unaided implanted ear[a] (AC & BC)		18.8
Unaided nonimplanted ear at least annually (AC & BC)		
Tympanometry, monaural (for cases of confuctive overlay)		3.4
Aided sound field thresholds (each implanted ear individually)		7.4
Hearing aid verification for nonimplanted ear		
Electroacoustic verification and real ear measures		22.0
Speech or speechlike stimulus at 60 dB SPL		
Aided speech recognition testing		
Recorded stimuli, 60 dB SPL, implant only and best-aided condition[a]		
CNC	One 50-item list	5–7
BKB-SIN test	One paired list	5–7
AzBio sentences	One 20-sentence list	5–7
If AzBio sentence recognition exceeds 60%, test at +10 dB SNR		
If AzBio sentence recognition at +10 dB SNR exceeds 60%, test at +5 dB SNR		
Administration of questionnaires (completed in waiting room prior to visit)		
Review pre-implant expectations questionnaire(s), as needed		
Post-implant administration of outcomes measures and quality-of-life questionnaire(s)		

AC air conduction; *BC* bone conduction; *CNC* consonant nucleus consonant; *SNR* signal-to-noise ratio

[a]Testing only in the nonimplanted ear should also be completed at least annually.

schedule (Fabry, Firszt, Gifford, Holden, & Koch, 2009). The recommendations included postoperative assessment of the MSTB—although not yet part of the MSTB at the time of publication—at 1, 3, 6, and 12 months, and annually thereafter. According to the recommendations, the implanted ear should be tested at each of these intervals; thus, for bilaterally implanted individuals who are implanted in the same surgical procedure, this would require testing the right, left, and bilateral conditions four times during the first year, which equals over 60 min of testing at each appointment. However, most adult bilateral recipients are implanted in sequential surgeries, in which case only the most recently implanted ear would have to be assessed at each visit during the first year.

Table 6–3 displays a modified testing schedule based on the Fabry et al. (2009) recommendations.

Table 6–3. Modified Postoperative Testing Schedule, for Adult Implant Recipients

Patient Group	1 month	3 months	6 months	12 months	Annually
Implanted ear alone	X	X	X	X	X
Nonimplanted ear (bimodal listeners)				X	X
"Best aided" (bimodal or bilateral cochlear implant)	X	X	X	X	X

Based on the recommendations of Fabry et al. (2009)

While some clinicians may be intimidated by the testing schedule, this does not represent a professional guideline or best-practices recommendation; it is simply an example of a testing schedule derived primarily from the recommendations of Fabry and colleagues (2009). As any seasoned clinician will attest, there are patient appointments for which we may plan to complete a full postoperative assessment, but complicated equipment issues, troubleshooting, and patient counseling, among other clinical issues, may arise. Though we have protocols in place to provide us with a framework by which we practice, the best clinicians know when to deviate from the protocol and/or testing schedule in order to better serve the needs of the patient.

Postoperative assessment is essential. Without it, we have no outcome measures on which to base the effectiveness of the intervention. For patients who have undergone an irreversible surgical procedure, it is even more critical to track postoperative performance longitudinally in order to assess the effectiveness of not just the surgery, but also our programming, the equipment, and the recommended rehabilitation strategy. Aided audiometric thresholds provide only a first-pass verification for our patients, but not unlike functional gain measures, aided sound-field thresholds provide information about tonal or noise-band detection. Detection estimates represent low-level processing that, even when optimal, does not necessarily equate one's *perception* of speech. As mentioned throughout this book, it is important for each cochlear implant program to determine its own protocol based on the goals

for both preoperative testing and postoperative assessment of speech understanding.

Another reason for completing regular postoperative testing is that these data are used in cases of device failure to confirm significant reduction in performance; thus, these data can help our patients obtain warranty replacement for internal device replacement. Though we do not like to think about device failures (and thankfully the percentage of failed devices is low, Eskander, Gordon, Kadhim, et al., 2011; Masterson, Kumar, Kong, et al., 2012; Roby, Ferrello, Huang, et al., 2012), failures do occur, and thus we must remain diligent in our documentation of patient outcomes over time.

Time Allotted for Postoperative Assessment

How much time should be allotted for postoperative assessment with adult implant recipients? This depends on the clinic protocol. Some clinics may choose to follow the full MSTB recommendations for select appointments but only include the minimum recommended testing schedule at most appointments due to time, space, and/or personnel restrictions. Other clinics may choose to incorporate the full MSTB recommendations but also obtain supplemental information, as obtained during the workup, including additional tests, questionnaires, and/or conditions. Using the MSTB's minimum recommended schedule as shown in Table 6–1, the approximate times for completion of each audiologic procedure were obtained from a time study of practice patterns for standard audiometry (Tucker, 2011) as well as for hearing aid verification (Busen & McCarthy, 2011). Time estimates for aided speech perception testing were obtained from the MSTB document itself. Table 6–2 provides time estimates for each of the procedures outlined in the MSTB. The estimates for audiometry and hearing aid verification reflect mean time estimates (in minutes) plus two standard deviations, as 95% of the expected values should fall within this range assuming a normal distribution. The time estimates for aided speech perception reflect the expected range of time (in minutes) needed for administration and scoring. Using the estimates provided in Table 6–2, the maximum estimated time required for aided sound-field threshold testing, hearing aid verification and aided speech perception testing for a bimodal patient (cochlear implant alone and the best aided condition) would range from 59 to 71 min. This time does not take into account the need to reprogram hearing aids should the patient's own hearing aid settings not be providing target audibility, nor does it include implant programming.

Although this may seem like a lot of time for testing, most postoperative assessments will not take a full 59 to 71 minutes; however, it is reasonable to err on the conservative side when allocating assessment time. The reason is that due to the severity of hearing loss and the highly individualized learning curve, not all patients will be able to communicate exclusively in an auditory/oral manner for the earliest postoperative periods. Thus, we may still need to provide written instructions on a large computer monitor facing the patient or have a standard set of simple written instructions for audiometry and speech perception testing that is often used at each cochlear implant evaluation.

SUBJECTIVE EVALUATION OF POSTOPERATIVE PERFORMANCE

As mentioned in Chapter 2, objective measures of postoperative speech perception performance and subjective assessments of perceived performance and/or benefit may not always be in good agreement with one another (Wackym, Runge-Samuelson, Firszt, Alkaf, & Burg, 2007). We have all experienced reports of terrible post-implant performance for patients demonstrating near ceiling-level performance. Conversely, we have also experienced reports of life-altering improvements in communication only to scratch our heads at the below-average performance observed in the test booth. A likely explanation for such discrepancies is that the laboratory-like conditions assessed in the audiometric test booth may not truly reflect real-world listening conditions; thus, it is important to utilize subjective assessment instruments that can help validate the efficacy of a particular treatment option, such as cochlear implantation. Clearly we recognize the efficacy of cochlear implantation with respect to restoration of audition—at least on a superficial, detection level—but we do not routinely assess the effect of cochlear implants on recipients' social and emotional welfare or the more global effects on quality of life. Furthermore, as noted in Chapter 2, we should be utilizing subjective assessment of communicative performance during the pre-implant workup; thus, the use of subjective measures during postoperative assessment provides patient-centered information that is not necessarily gauged with standardized clinical measures of speech recognition. (See Chapter 2 for a detailed discussion of the available validated instruments.)

In addition to the validated questionnaires designed to track outcome measures and overall quality-of-life changes resulting from cochlear implantation, Chapter 2 also discusses the use of preoperative expectations questionnaires. Pre-implant expectation questionnaires allow patients to document, in writing, what they believe cochlear implants can provide for them in terms of benefit. It is not standard clinical practice to review the preoperative expectations questionnaire during postoperative assessment; however, for those patients expressing frustration regarding progress or exhibiting unrealistic expectations, review of the preoperative questionnaire serves as an excellent counseling tool, particularly for those patients expressing expectations that may differ from their own written pre-implant responses.

ROLE OF THE SOCIAL WORKER AND/OR PSYCHOLOGIST IN POSTOPERATIVE ASSESSMENT AND MANAGEMENT

As mentioned in the previous section, postoperative questionnaire data can provide useful information into the overall social and emotional well-being of our patients; thus, another clinical use of the postoperative questionnaire data includes identifying those individuals who may be having considerable difficulty adjusting to the cochlear implant and/or exhibiting highly unrealistic expectations despite having "passed" the preoperative candidacy workup. This information may prove useful to the cochlear implant team in order for the surgeon to make a psychological/psychiatric referral.

We often associate preoperative patients as being those most likely to suffer the psychosocial effects of hearing loss including increased incidence of depression, social anxiety, loneliness, and overall psychological distress (e.g., Nachtegaal et al., 2009; Gopinath et al., 2009; Knutson, Johnson, & Murray, 2006; Abrams, Barnett, Hoth, Schultz, & Kaboli, 2006). Although cochlear implantation has been shown to significantly reduce depression and other psychosocial symptoms in individuals with hearing loss (Knutson et al., 1991, 1998; Olze et al., 2011; Poissant, Beaudoin, Huang, Brodsky, & Lee, 2008), there are still some psychological risks associated with cochlear implantation that may require postoperative referral and clinical management. Studies have shown that spouses of individuals with hearing loss exhibit elevated levels of psychological stress and anxiety (Hetu, Lalonde, & Getty, 1987; Hetu, Riverin, Lalande, Getty, & St-Cyr, 1988; Lormore & Stephens, 1994; Brooks, Hallam, & Mellor, 2001; Piercy & Piercy, 2002; Knutson et al., 2006; Scarinci, Worrall, & Hickson, 2008); thus, it is possible that should an implant recipient not make rapid or expected progress following surgery, the level of stress within the marital relationship may also be elevated. On the other end of the spectrum, there have been reports of high-performing patients achieving increased independence and confidence, which also has the potential to affect one's marital relationship.

Although these are issues clearly outside the scope of audiology, speech/language pathology, and otolaryngology, our patients often confide in us as trusted professionals, and thus these are issues about which we should be aware.

MEDICAL AND SURGICAL MANAGEMENT OF THE ADULT IMPLANT RECIPIENT

The cochlear implant surgeon, a specialist in otology or neuro-otology, plays an obviously critical role in the preoperative determination of implant candidacy. Otologists also play a critical role in the *postoperative* management of implant recipients. It is customary for surgeons to see implant patients around the time of the initial activation for postoperative check of incision, scalp flap, and reconciliation of surgically related symptoms (such as dizziness, taste disturbances, pain, etc.). This postoperative check, however, does not mark the end of the surgeon's management of the implant patient. The otologist and his or her medical team will also ensure that all cochlear implant candidates are up to date on their immunizations not only prior to cochlear implantation but also over time as the Centers for Disease Control updates the recommended booster protocol for age-specific pneumococcal vaccinations.

From an insurance-coverage perspective, Medicare requires patients to obtain a physician order for audiologic follow-up and programming. In order for the physician to be in compliance, he or she needs to maintain medical oversight of a patient's care. Notwithstanding the insurance requirement for a signed physician order for regular audiologic management, implant recipients remain under the medical care of their implanting surgeons and should thus be seen regularly for otoscopic and postauricular evaluation. Many otologists continue to see their adult implant patients on an annual or biennial basis as standard practice. In addition to this standard practice, audiologists are undoubtedly closely acquainted with the overall otoscopic and postauricular health of implant patients and refer them for medical consultation in cases of redness, irritation, skin breakdown, electrode/device extrusion, or any other physical concern related to the implant that is outside the audiologist's scope of practice.

CONCLUSION

Postoperative assessment of outcomes is an essential component of the best-practices management for adult implant recipients. Postoperative assessment is not limited to patient-history taking regarding how well a patient thinks he or she is doing. This is standard practice for too many implant programs. Without comprehensive and frequent assessment of outcomes, including speech recognition, aided audiometric thresholds, and subjective perception of benefit and quality of life, we are not engaging in evidence-based practices. Our patients undergo an irreversible surgical procedure, and although they often sing the praises of their implants, we simply cannot provide our best programming and management without verifying our efforts. We do not need to provide our services for free because there are billable codes for postoperative assessment including CPT 92626, which can be used alone or with the 59 modifier when completing implant programming during the same appointment.

A recurrent theme of this book is that each implant program and team develops and refines its own protocols with respect to pre- and post-implant assessment of patient performance. Though there are guidelines, such as the MSTB, each program has its own unique needs, patients, and culture. More important than the actual protocol is *adherence* to the protocol in order for the team to generate program-specific norms and for the longitudinal assessment of patient performance. Postoperative data obtained over the long term provides valuable clinical information about variability in patient performance, need for programming adjustments, equipment malfunction, etc. It is expected that over time the individual metrics used in the protocol will change just as we have seen the evolution of the MSTB over the past two decades. We will be ready for these changes and will be able to document the relation-ship between patient performance on previous metrics with future metrics as long as we adhere to our protocols for postoperative assessment of performance.

REFERENCES

Abrams, T. E., Barnett, M. J., Hoth, A., Schultz, S., & Kaboli, P. J. (2006). The relationship between hearing impairment and depression in older veterans. *Journal of the American Geriatric Society, 54*(9), 1475–1477.

ANSI. (2004, R2009). Methods for Manual Pure-Tone Threshold Audiometry. American National Standards Institute, S3.21-2004, New York, NY.

Carlson, M. C., Driscoll, C. L. W., Gifford, R. H., Service, G., Tombers, N., Hughes-Borst, R., et al. (2011). Implications of minimizing trauma during conventional length cochlear implantation. *Otology & Neurotology, 32*(6), 962–968.

Brooks, D. N., Hallam, R. S., & Mellor, P. A. (2001). The effects on significant others of providing a hearing aid to the hearing-impaired partner. *British Journal of Audiology, 35*, 165–171.

Busen, J., & McCarthy, P. (2011). *Probe-microphone measurements: Commonly used or neglected?* San Diego, CA: AudiologyNOW!.

Eskander, A., Gordon, K. A., Kadhim, L., Papaioannou, V., Cushing, S. L., James, A. L., & Papsin, B. C. (2011). Low pediatric cochlear implant failure rate: contributing factors in large-volume practice. *Archives of Otolaryngology–Head Neck Surgery, 137*, 1190–1196.

Etymotic Research, Inc. (2005). BKB-SIN test. Speech-in-Noise Test, version 1.03. Retrieved from http://www.etymotic.com

Fabry, D., Firszt, J. B., Gifford, R. H., Holden, L. K., & Koch, D. (2009). Evaluating speech perception benefit in adult cochlear implant recipients. *Audiology Today, 21*, 37–42.

Gantz, B. J., Hansen, M. R., Turner, C. W., Oleson, J. J., Reiss, L. A., & Parkinson, A. J. (2009). Hybrid 10 clinical trial: Preliminary results. *Audiology and Neurotology, 14*(Suppl 1), 32–38.

Gopinath, B., Wang, J. J., Schneider, J., Burlutsky, G., Snowdon, J., McMahon, C. M., et al. (2009). Depressive symptoms in older adults with hearing impairments: The Blue Mountains Study. *Journal of the American Geriatric Society, 57*(7), 1306–1308.

Gstoettner, W. K., van de Heyning, P., O'Connor, A. F., Morera, C., Sainz, M., Vermeire, K., et al. (2008).

Electric acoustic stimulation of the auditory system: Results of a multi-centre investigation. *Acta Oto-Laryngologica, 128,* 968–975.

Hetu, R., Lalonde, M., & Getty, L. (1987). Psychosocial disadvantages associated with occupational hearing loss as experienced in the family. *Audiology, 26,* 141–152.

Hetu, R., Riverin, L., Lalande, N., Getty, L., & St-Cyr, C. (1988). Qualitative analysis of the handicap associated with occupational hearing loss. *British Journal of Audiology, 22,* 251–264.

ISO 8253-2. (1998). Acoustics—audiometric test methods, part 2: Sound field audiometry with pure tone and narrow-band test signals. International Organization for Standardization.

Killion, M., Niquette, P., Revit, L., & Skinner, M. (2001). Quick SIN and BKB-SIN, two new speech-in-noise tests permitting SNR-50 estimates in 1 to 2 min (A). *Journal of the Acoustical Society of America, 109*(5), 2502–2512.

Knutson, J. F., Johnson, A., & Murray, K. T. (2006). Social and emotional characteristics of adults seeking a cochlear implant and their spouses. *British Journal of Health Psychology, 11*(Pt 2), 279–292.

Knutson, J. F., Murray, K. T., Husarek, S., Westerhouse, K., Woodworth, G., Gantz, B. J., & Tyler, R. S. (1998). Psychological change over 54 months of cochlear implant use. *Ear and Hearing, 19,* 191–201.

Knutson, J. F., Schartz, H. A., Gantz, B. J., Tyler, R. S., Hinrichs, J. V., & Woodworth, G. (1991). Psychological change following 18 months of cochlear implant use. *Annals of Otology, Rhinology and Laryngology, 110,* 877–882.

Lormore, K. A., & Stephens, S. D. (1994) Use of the open-ended questionnaire with patients and their significant others. *British Journal of Audiology, 28,* 81–89.

Mackersie, C. L. (2002). Tests of speech perception abilities. *Current Opinion in Otolaryngology & Head and Neck Surgery, 10,* 392–397.

Masterson, L., Kumar, S., Kong, J. H., Briggs, L., Donnelly, N. Axon, P. R., & Gray, R. F. (2012). Cochlear implant failures: lessons learned from a UK centre. *Journal of Laryngology and Otology, 126*(1), 15–21.

Nachtegaal, J., Smit, J. H., Smits, C., Bezemer, P. D., van Beek, J. H., Festen, J. M., et al. (2009). The association between hearing status and psychosocial health before the age of 70 years: Results from an Internet-based national survey on hearing. *Ear and Hearing, 30*(3), 302–312.

Nilsson, M., Soli, S., & Sullivan J. (1994). Development of the Hearing in Noise test for the measurement of speech reception thresholds in quiet and in noise. *Journal of the Acoustical Society of America, 95,* 1085–1099.

Olze, H., Szczepek, A. J., Haupt, H., Förster, U., Zirke, N., Gräbel, S., et al. (2011). Cochlear implantation has a positive influence on quality of life, tinnitus, and psychological comorbidity. 2011. *Laryngoscope, 121*(10), 2220–2227.

Peterson, G. E., & Lehiste, I. (1962). Revised CNC lists for auditory tests. *Journal of Speech and Hearing Disorders, 27,* 62–72.

Piercy, S. K., & Piercy, F. P. (2002) Couple dynamics and attributions when one partner has an acquired hearing loss: Implications for couple therapy. *Journal of Marital and Family Therapy, 28*(3), 315–326.

Poissant, S. F., Beaudoin, F., Huang, J., Brodsky, J., & Lee, D. J. (2008). Impact of cochlear implantation on speech understanding, depression, and loneliness in the elderly. *Journal of Otolaryngology—Head and Neck Surgery, 37*(4), 488–494.

Roby, B. B., Ferrello, M., Huang, T. C., Rimell, F. L., & Levine, S. C. (2012). Symptom timeline preceding cochlear implant failure: An institutional experience. *Otolaryngology—Head and Neck Surgery, 146*(5), 782–787.

Scarinci, N., Worrall, L., & Hickson, L. (2008). The effect of hearing impairment in older people on the spouse. *International Journal of Audiology, 47,* 141–151.

Silverman, S. R., & Hirsch, I. J. (1955). Problems related to the use of speech in clinical audiometry. *Annals of Otology, Rhinology and Laryngology, 64,* 1234–1244.

Skarzynski, H., Lorens, A., Piotrowska, A., & Anderson, I. (2006). Partial deafness cochlear implantation provides benefit to a new population of individuals with hearing loss. *Acta Oto-Laryngologica, 126,* 934–940.

Skinner, M., Fourakis, M. S., Holden, T. A., Holden, L., & Demorest, M. E. (1999). Identification of speech by cochlear implant recipients with the Multipeak (MPEAK) and Spectral Peak (SPEAK) speech coding strategies II. Consonants. *Ear and Hearing, 20,* 443–460.

Skinner, M. W., Holden, L. K., Holden, T. A., Demorest, M. E., & Fourakis, M. S. (1997). Speech recognition at simulated soft, conversational, and raised-to-loud vocal efforts by adults with cochlear implants. *Journal of the Acoustical Society of America, 101*(6), 3766–3782.

Spahr, A. J., Dorman, M. F., Litvak, L. L., Van Wie, S., Gifford, R. H., Loizou, P. C., et al. (2012). Development and validation of the AzBio Sentence Lists. *Ear and Hearing, 33,* 112–117.

Tucker, M. (2001). *A time study of audiological practice patterns and the impact of reimbursement changes from third party payers.* Theses and dissertations. Paper 1543.

Retrieved from http://scholarcommons.usf.edu/etd/1543

Valente, M., Abrams, H., Benson, D., Chisolm, T., Citron, D., Hampton, D., et al. (2006). Guidelines for the audiologic management of adult hearing impairment. *Audiology Today, 18*(5), 32–36.

Wackym, P. A., Runge-Samuelson, C. L., Firszt, J. B., Alkaf, F. M., & Burg, L. S. (2007). More challenging speech perception tasks demonstrate binaural benefit in bilateral cochlear implant users. *Ear and Hearing, 28*, 80S–85S.

||| 7 |||

Elements of Postoperative Assessment: Pediatric Implant Recipients

René H. Gifford

Protocols for evaluating the postoperative performance of pediatric implant recipients are as fluid as a child's interest. This is particularly true for the youngest patients. As discussed in Chapter 6, the ideal speech perception test should be reliable, sensitive to differences between listening/testing conditions, and correlate with real world speech understanding (Mackersie, 2002). The biggest obstacle for postoperative management of pediatric implant patients is the gathering of information from a child who is pre- or peri-verbal. Although this is challenging, it is not impossible and should remain a central goal of each audiologic programming visit. It is our role as clinicians to ensure that a child's amplification—whether it be with cochlear implants and/or hearing aids—is appropriate and that the amplification is maximizing his or her auditory potential. Thus there are many fac-

tors to be considered, other than just the *exact measures* to be used, in the postoperative assessment of pediatric implant recipients.

POST-IMPLANT AUDIOLOGIC EVALUATION

Cochlear Implant "Aided" Audiometric Thresholds

Given that cochlear implants provide transcutaneous transmission via radio-frequency signals, the physical output level cannot be directly measured as is the case with hearing aids. We can, however, still estimate the minimum audibility levels for a child's implant map (Figure 7–1). As discussed in Chapter 6, Skinner and colleagues (1997, 1999) discussed the function of sound-field audiometric thresholds for determining the minimum audibility available for implant recipients. It is considered

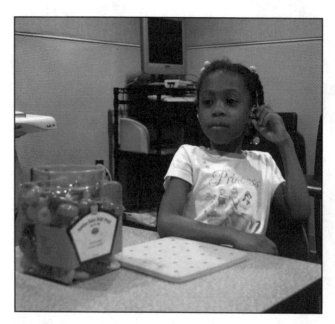

FIGURE 7–1. Shown here is a 6-year old girl engaging in conditioned play audiometry to assess postoperative audiometric detection thresholds with her cochlear implant.

standard practice to optimize cochlear implant mapping to achieve aided sound-field thresholds in the range of 20 to 25 dB HL (for 250 to 6000 Hz) for pediatric implant recipients (with 20 to 30 dB HL generally being acceptable for adult recipients). For children with bilateral implants, aided sound-field thresholds should be obtained individually for each ear so as to allow for individual-ear-map optimization.

Documenting sound-field thresholds in the range of 20 to 25 dB HL provides assurance of audibility for low-level stimuli, such as soft speech (e.g., Skinner et al., 1997). The reason is that "soft" speech levels are in the range of 45 to 50 dB SPL (Pearsons, Bennett, & Fidell, 1977), which puts phonemic content of soft speech as low as 15 dB HL (e.g., Mueller & Killion, 1990). Given that children are actively acquiring speech and language via implant sound processors, it is considered more critical to achieve audibility for various levels of speech than even for adult implant recipients. As stated in the American Academy of Audiology's Pediatric Amplification Protocol (2003), "the primary goal is audibility of speech regardless of input level or vocal effort." We must be wary, however, that sound-field thresholds

below 15 dB HL are problematic, because we are introducing considerable noise to the input dynamic range and increasing the likelihood of audible circuit noise. Lower thresholds are not necessarily better when it comes to optimizing audibility for our pediatric implant recipients; 20 to 25 dB HL remains the goal, with an occasional threshold at 15 dB HL also being acceptable.

Microphone Listening Check

Another important note is that although aided sound-field thresholds provide verification of implant mapping for low-level inputs, there is no substitution for a listening check of the sound-processor microphone. Pediatric audiologists routinely listen to implant processor microphones to check for low-level humming, static, or any variation of compromised sound quality. Although we recommend that parents and educators routinely listen to the microphone of the sound processor(s), we should not rely solely on parental report as clinicians simply have more experience listening to microphones and are thus more attuned to slight deviations from normal. Microphone listening checks remains a low-tech yet highly important tool for postoperative assessment of performance.

Calibration and Test Conditions

Table 6–1 in Chapter 6 displays frequency-specific correction factors for sound-field threshold estimation referencing a 0° azimuth calibration. (See Chapter 6 for additional detailed information regarding issues central to sound-field calibration for aided sound-field thresholds.)

Stimulus for Testing: Frequency-Modulated Tones and Narrow-Band Noise

As discussed in Chapter 6, sound-field thresholds are obtained with both frequency-modulated (FM) or warbled tones and narrow-band noise. All pediatric audiologists are aware of the need for FM tones in the sound field to avoid problems associated with standing waves; however, clinicians are not necessarily aware of problems associated with the use of narrow-band noise for threshold estimation in the sound field. Audiometers will always be calibrated for narrow-band noise presentation via headphones or insert earphones as used for effective masking levels. Not all acoustic engineers will routinely calibrate audiometers for narrow-band noise presentation in the free field. As mentioned in Chapter 6, computer-based audiometers utilizie narrower-band noise that was designed specifically for threshold estimation and sound-field audiometry. This narrower-band noise is created with much steeper filter slopes which affords accurate, frequency-specific thresholds.

Assessment of Acoustic Hearing Status

Implanted Ear

As mentioned in Chapters 2 and 6, otologists, audiologists, and even patients are increasingly aware of the possibilities of hearing preservation with cochlear implantation (e.g., Gstoettner et al., 2008; Gantz et al., 2009; Carlson et al., 2011; Skarzynski, Lorens, Piotrowska, & Anderson, 2006). Hearing preservation is not limited to adult implant recipients. In fact, children with residual low-frequency hearing are being implanted at increasing rates, particularly for those children with precipitously sloping hearing losses who are not making auditory progress with appropriately fitted hearing aids (e.g., Ha, Wood, Krishnaswamy, & Rajan, 2012; Kuthubutheen, Hedne, Krishnaswamy, & Rajan, 2012; Jayawardena, Kuthubutheen, & Rajan, 2012; Skarzynski & Lorens, 2010; Brown, Hullar, Cadieux, & Chole, 2010; Skarzynski, Lorens, D'Haese, Walkowiak, Piotrowska, Sliwa & Anderson, 2002). Pediatric implant recipients with considerable low-frequency acoustic hearing tend to be older than the typical pediatric implant recipient, and thus assessment of postoperative preserved hearing is generally possible, even at the initial activation appointment.

If possible, it is recommended that unaided hearing be checked at the initial activation appointment, or shortly thereafter. Both air conduction and bone conduction thresholds are required to adequately assess residual acoustic hearing status. Because residual blood and/or fluid may be present in the middle ear space (from the surgery), otoscopy and also possibly tympanograms may be completed; however, as discussed in Chapter 6 for adult recipients, it is highly recommended that the audiology team discuss this with the surgeon to gain medical clearance for tympanometry following surgery (particularly for initial activations occurring sooner than 2 weeks after surgery).

Should acoustic hearing be present following surgery, we will continue to monitor this hearing longitudinally. Given that there will potentially be a large proportion of young implant recipients for whom postoperative assessment of preserved hearing is not possible at the initial activation appointment, it will be important to obtain pure-tone thresholds in the implanted at a follow-up appointment—preferably during the first few months following surgery. One may question the utility of assessing hearing preservation for the implanted ear, because we will likely not consider fitting an in-the-ear (ITE) hearing aid in the ear of a pediatric implant recipient; however, sound processors with integrated hearing aid circuitry are already commercially available in Europe and Canada and will be available in the United States in the near future. Having the knowledge of preserved hearing for our patient population will be the first step in electroacoustic management once such technology becomes readily available.

Of course, there will be many pediatric implant recipients who have little-to-no acoustic hearing prior to surgery. For these children, it is not as critical to assess postoperative hearing status. Nonetheless, there are reports documenting the need for "structural" preservation with cochlear implantation as minimally traumatic surgical techniques may yield higher levels of postoperative performance (e.g., Gantz, Dunn, Walker, Kenworthy, Van Voorst, Tomblin & Turner, 2010; Carlson et al., 2011).

Nonimplanted Ear (Bimodal Listeners)

For our bimodal patients, we will continue to manage the hearing and associated effectiveness and appropriateness of amplification in the nonimplanted ear. Pediatric audiologists already do a great job of managing the whole child—including the hearing aid *and* cochlear implant—for bimodal children; however, it remains tempting to focus almost entirely on the implanted ear such that the nonimplanted ear is neglected. We must not forget that in order to assess the effectiveness of the hearing modality in the child's speech/language development and speech understanding, we must ensure that we are truly assessing the best-aided condition. Thus, even for the youngest patients, we should be completing (1) regular pure-tone audiometry, whether it be via visual reinforcement audiometry, conditioned play audiometry, or conventional audiometry for older children, and (2) probe-microphone measurements to verify hearing aid settings.

As discussed in Chapter 3 with pre-implant protocols, according to the American Academy of Audiology's Pediatric Amplification Protocol (2003), best practices dictate that hearing aids must be verified using either probe-microphone measurements or test-box verification with patient-specific real ear to coupler difference (RECD) corrections. Given that many children will be fitted with nonlinear hearing aid circuitry, a prescriptive fitting formula such as DSL m[i/o] (Seewald, Ross, & Spiro, 1985; Cornelisse, Seewald, & Jamieson, 1995; Scollie et al., 2005) is recommended in order to verify audibility at various input levels (see Chapter 3 for further detail). Note that the RECD should be measured every time the child has an earmold change and/or any time there is a change in middle ear status. For older children who are not getting earmold remakes as often as younger children and infants, RECD measures should be repeated on an annual basis to coincide with the annual hearing assessment.

As discussed in Chapter 6 in reference to adult postoperative assessment, it is important that clinicians not substitute functional gain measures for probe-microphone measurements with bimodal patients. Functional gain may appear tempting given that we will already be heading to the sound booth for aided implant thresholds and parents may even request that hearing aid thresholds be placed on the audiogram. Functional gain measures do not verify hearing aid settings in reference to aided audibility nor do they provide information regarding the input/output characteristics of hearing aids. If one wants to obtain functional gain measurements with the implant and hearing aid individually, as long as functional gain is not substituted for real ear measures, this may be viewed as a counseling tool and to explain the differences in verification techniques across implants and hearing aids to the child's family.

ASSESSMENT OF SPEECH RECOGNITION ABILITIES

Recorded Materials

A central component of postoperative assessment for pediatric cochlear implant recipients for older children involves the behavioral assessment of speech recognition. Many children with hearing loss may continue to rely heavily on visual cues such as lip reading and more global nonverbal communication; thus, in order to gain an understanding of a child's auditory-based understanding—and more importantly, to ensure that we are maximizing auditory/oral speech understanding—recorded speech stimuli are presented without visual cues.

A critical aspect of speech recognition testing for older children involves the use of recorded speech materials. As shown in Chapter 2, Figure 2–1, the variability associated with monitored live voice (MLV) presentation does not lend itself well to the accurate assessment of postoperative outcomes. Despite the variability and associated problems with assessing speech recognition via MLV, depending on a child's age and/or global developmental status, MLV may be required to elicit reliable responses; however, MLV administration of speech stimuli is not appropriate for longitudinal assessment of postoperative performance. (See Chapter 2 for detailed information regarding calibration of recorded stimuli for presentation in the sound field.)

Presentation Levels

An important aspect of postoperative speech recognition testing involves the presentation levels of the recorded speech stimuli. As discussed in Chapters 2 and 3, 60 dBA represents average conversational-level speech, and thus it should be considered the *highest* presentation level used for assessment of postoperative outcomes. Many clinics also routinely use a lower presentation level for both adults and children given that average, casual speech levels for children and women range from 50 to 56 dBA (see Chapter 3, Table 3–1) (Pearsons et al., 1977; Olsen, 1998).

Many clinicians inquire about the HL dial setting required to achieve 50 or 60 dB SPL (A weighted; see Chapter 2) in the sound booth. The answer depends completely on the material used, the source of the material, the distance between the loudspeaker and the listener, the size of the room, as well as a number of other variables. (See Chapter 2 for a detailed description on the calibration of speech stimuli for presentation in the sound field to achieve set SPL levels for testing.)

Multiple Estimates of Speech Recognition

Unlike postoperative follow-up for adult patients, pediatric implant recipients tend to be seen more frequently for routine mapping and assessment. Multiple visits provide us with frequent opportunities to not only optimize mapping but also to assess postoperative outcomes for audibility and speech recognition. There are not currently any recommended guidelines for the frequency of postoperative assessment for pediatric implant recipients. Until such guidelines are determined, it remains the responsibility of each implant team to determine its own protocol dictating the number of postoperative audiologic assessments that should take place, or should at least be attempted, during the postoperative period.

Speech-Perception Metrics

Adult implant audiologists have the Minimum Speech Test Battery (MSTB) as a best-practices guideline for the administration and assessment of speech recognition. Unfortunately, there is not yet a pediatric version of the MSTB from which we can determine our individual clinic protocols. As discussed throughout this book, more important than the individual protocol and metrics

themselves is that all clinicians at an implant center follow the same protocol.

Assessing postoperative speech recognition for pediatric implant patients should be undertaken on a metric-by-metric basis, as we can never be certain how long a child will remain a cooperative participant. For this reason it is recommended that each clinic develop a "priority protocol" for assessing speech recognition at each visit. A priority protocol specifies not only the metrics to be used but also the order of administration. This means that if time allows for only one test to be completed, the same test or test category would be completed for all patients regardless of age, development, or clinician. If additional time is available and the child's level of cooperation affords further testing, the next metric in the priority protocol would be administered. This way, at a very minimum, a cochlear implant program would have the same information from each child, even if only a single metric could be administered.

Figure 7–2 displays a sample priority protocol for pediatric speech recognition testing. The priority of metrics progresses from left to right with (1) auditory discrimination, (2) word recognition, (3) sentence recognition in quiet, and then (4) sentence recognition in noise being prioritized for any given listening condition being assessed. Within a given category, a clinician would begin with the developmentally appropriate metric. For example, if you have been following a child over time and know that she is capable of completing open-set word testing, then there would be no need to begin with auditory discrimination tasks or closed-set measures. Despite being a waste of precious assessment time, any information gleaned would be completely inconsistent with the child's realistic auditory capabilities and runs the risk of inflating the child's performance. On the other end of the spectrum, if you have a patient with limited auditory skills, delayed development, and who has never been administered closed-set measures, then it would be a futile effort to first attempt speech recognition assessment using a difficult metric such as PB-K or CNC monosyllables. The sample priority protocol shown in Figure 7–2 should be used as a guideline and not as the standard for pediatric speech testing, because there is currently no consensus on a pediatric minimum speech test battery.

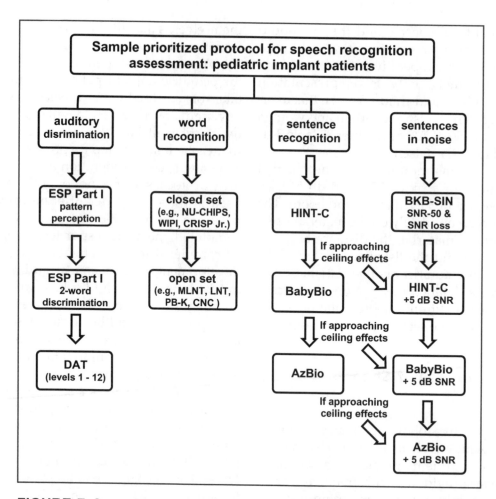

FIGURE 7–2. Sample priority protocol for speech recognition testing in pediatric implant recipients. **ESP** Early Speech Perception; **DAT** Discrimination After Training; **HINT-C** Hearing-in-Noise Test for Children; **WIPI** Word Identification Picture Intelligibility; **CRISP** Children's Realistic Intelligibility of Speech Perception; **NU-CHIPS** Northwestern University Children's Perception of Speech; **LNT** Lexical Neighborhood Test; **MLNT** Multisyllabic Lexical Neighborhood Test; **CNC** Consonant Nucleus Consonant.

As shown in Figure 7–2 there are *nonspeech* measures that may be used for postoperative assessment of children with limited skills for which assessment of auditory discrimination/detection may be the goal. Part I of the Early Speech Perception (ESP) test (Geers & Moog, 1989) includes pattern perception and two-word identification. Another nonspeech measure is the Discrimination After Training (DAT) (Thielmeir, 1982) test, which evaluates detection of speech as well as temporal-based cues such as duration and timing discrimination; thus, there are viable nonspeech measures for use with our youngest

patients and those patients with lower auditory skills and development. We may first begin with pattern-perception testing rather than jumping into a closed-set measure of word recognition, though this decision is often made on a patient-by-patient basis.

Pediatric Measures of Word and Sentence Recognition

For a detailed description of available word and sentence metrics for pediatric clinical use, please see Chapter 3.

Testing Conditions

The testing conditions to be assessed in the postoperative assessment period vary depending on the goal of the appointment. Individual ear assessment is desired for all implanted ears to ensure optimal audibility and speech recognition abilities for each implanted ear; however, because children are rarely listening in a single-ear condition, except during therapy sessions, assessing the best-aided condition also makes practical sense. As mentioned throughout this chapter, there is not yet a pediatric MSTB with which to guide our protocol for the listening conditions to be assessed; thus, professional clinical judgment is vital to guide the assessment visit. For example, if the goal of the appointment is to determine whether a second implant should be considered, then individual ear performance as well as the bimodal condition would provide the greatest utility. In another example, if a child recently obtained a second implant, then it would likely be the goal of the assessment to characterize performance for the newly implanted ear, and if time allowed, the bilateral condition. Because children may not remain cooperative throughout the entire testing session, it will likely take multiple visits, sometimes over months to years, to obtain a complete audiologic profile of postoperative speech understanding performance.

Developing a Postoperative Protocol

Developing a postoperative speech understanding protocol is an important task for each cochlear implant program. As counseled by Madell (2010), the purpose of speech recognition testing is not to allow the child to obtain the best possible score. Rather, our goal should be to assess the effectiveness of the chosen habilitation strategy (conventional amplification versus cochlear implants), hearing modality (bimodal versus bilateral), as well as evaluating the efficacy of the current technology settings. Furthermore, we should be able to use the information gathered from postoperative speech recognition testing to guide future habilitation, recommendations for scheduling of subsequent follow-up visits, programming modifications, as well as assisting educational recommendations such as technologic needs in the classroom.

An important point with respect to the recommended conditions to be included in a postoperative protocol is that children are rarely in quiet listening environments. As discussed in Chapter 3, educational acoustic research has shown that occupied classroom noise can range from 48 to 69 dBA with the mean level approximately 65 dBA for an early elementary classroom (e.g., Sanders, 1965; Nober & Nober, 1975; Bess, Sinclair, & Riggs, 1984; Finitzo-Hieber, 1988). In fact, educational acoustic research has shown that Leq 24-hr measurement averages 87.3 dBA for all school-age children and 95.5 dBA for fifth graders (Clark & Govett, 1995). Clearly a child's everyday listening environment is much noisier than that encountered by the typical adult; thus it follows that postoperative assessment of speech understanding should include speech-in-noise testing. Without speech-in-noise testing, we cannot fully assess a child's auditory capabilities in his typical everyday listening environment and as a consequence, may be grossly overestimating performance.

Parental Questionnaires for Assessing Postoperative Development of Auditory Skills

Auditory skills development for younger children will most likely be gauged via auditory questionnaire data, parental report, and speech/language assessment. This is particularly true for the youngest implant recipients (<12 months up to 2 years of age) for which immediate postoperative assessment of speech understanding is not possible using conventional metrics as displayed in Figure 7–2. For a detailed description of the most widely used pediatric auditory questionnaires, see Table 3–2 in Chapter 3. It is recommended that, regardless of the progress made immediately postactivation, we administer the same questionnaires that were administered immediately pre-implant so that we are able to describe the relative benefit derived from cochlear implantation in a pre- versus post-implant comparison.

ROLE OF THE SOCIAL WORKER AND/OR PSYCHOLOGIST IN THE POSTOPERATIVE PERIOD

The role of the social worker and/or psychologist in the postoperative period tends to be less critical than that experienced preoperatively. Social workers are able to provide counseling and support for families in terms of finances as related to medical care surrounding aural habilitation, particularly if insurance restrictions arise. Families may be unaware of the financial resources available to them for insurance coverage of medical care, therapy, and assistive listening devices. Social workers not only provide this information but also help provide access to the appropriate paperwork and help families navigate through the application processes. In some cases, social workers can help coordinate medical and therapy appointments as well as review the past and current schedule of appointments to ensure that all medical specialties and evaluations have been made available to the family.

Psychological evaluations may come into play during the postoperative period for those families of children not making expected auditory progress following implantation. For children implanted as infants and young toddlers, any future issues surrounding developmental delay may not yet be known at the time of implantation; thus, should a child fail to make expected post-implant progress despite adherence to the recommended therapy schedule and full-time usage of the implant (i.e., wearing the sound processor during all waking hours), developmental psychological evaluation may be recommended by the cochlear implant team.

MEDICAL AND SURGICAL MANAGEMENT OF THE PEDIATRIC IMPLANT RECIPIENT

The cochlear implant surgeon plays a vital role in the *postoperative* management of all implant recipients—especially pediatric recipients. For a detailed description of the surgeon's role in postoperative care, see Chapter 6.

Most insurance plans will require patients to obtain a physician order for audiologic and speech/language follow-up and programming. In order for the physician to be in compliance, he or she needs to maintain medical oversight of a patient's care. Notwithstanding the insurance requirement for a signed physician order for regular audiologic management, implant recipients remain under the medical care of their implanting surgeons and should thus be seen regularly for otoscopic and postauricular evaluation. Many otologists continue to see their pediatric implant patients on an annual or biennial basis as standard practice.

CONCLUSION

Cochlear implants have the potential to change the course of a child's life allowing for normal to near-normal development of speech, language, and literacy. Even for those children not able to achieve an auditory/oral approach to speech and language, cochlear implants provide sound awareness increasing safety and quality of life for the recipient. In order to do our part and ensure that the audiologic management of the technology is providing the child with the highest auditory potential, we must diligently seek to assess post-operative performance for audibility, auditory-skills progress, as well as speech-understanding skills. (See Chapter 8 for further information regarding the aspects of postoperative assessment related to the speech/language pathologist [SLP], auditory verbal therapist [AVT], and deaf educator.) The interdisciplinary cochlear implant team offers patients the highest level of care needed to excel and progress through the postoperative process. As has been mentioned previously, obtaining cochlear implants is only the first step in the journey, as the hardest work occurs *after* the surgery.

Postoperative assessment of outcomes is a vital component of the best-practices management for implant audiologists working with children. Postoperative assessment is not limited to auditory questionnaire data or obtaining speech and language records from the child's SLP, AVT, and deaf educator. Audiologists, SLPs, AVTs, and deaf educators must make a concerted effort to work as a management "team" to provide a child with the best chances for maximizing his auditory potential. Caraway (2012) uses the term *flexible team boundaries* to describe a team-building approach for a child's audiologist, SLP/AVT, and deaf educator to integrate the management of a child's technology, therapy schedule, habilitation options, and educational-placement recommendations. We are all working toward the same goal but often fail to work together perhaps simply because we work in different physical locations.

Each cochlear implant center has its own needs, patients, and culture; thus, it is up to each individual center and its team members to develop a pediatric protocol for postoperative assessment and to define its team boundaries for patient management. More important than the actual protocol is *adherence* to the protocol in order for the team to generate program-specific norms and for the longitudinal assessment of patient performance. Postoperative data obtained over the long term will provide us with valuable clinical information regarding variability in patient performance, need for programming adjustments, equipment malfunction, etc. It is a given that over time the individual metrics used in the protocol will change just as we have seen the evolution of the adult MSTB over the past two decades and as new pediatric measures are developed for the evolving population of pediatric implant recipients. We will be ready for evolutionary changes and able to document the relationship between patient performance on previous measures with future measures only if we adhere to our current protocols for postoperative assessment of performance.

REFERENCES

American Academy of Audiology. (2003). Pediatric amplification protocol. Retrieved July 20, 2012, from http://www.audiology.org

Bess, F. H., Sinclair, J. S., & Riggs, D. (1984). Group amplification in schools for the hearing impaired. *Ear and Hearing, 5*, 138–144.

Brown, R. F., Hullar, T. E., Cadieux, J. H., & Chole, R. A. (2010). Residual hearing preservation after pediatric cochlear implantation. *Otology & Neurotology, 31*(8), 1221–1226.

Caraway, T. (2012). Play it by ear: Strategies and techniques to improve outcomes for children with hearing loss. *Controversial issues in pediatric audiology.* New York, NY: A. G. Bell.

Carlson, M. C., Driscoll, C. L. W., Gifford, R. H., Service, G., Tombers, N., Hughes-Borst, R., et al. (2011). Implications of minimizing trauma during conventional length cochlear implantation. *Otology & Neurotology, 32*, 962–968.

Clark, W. W., & Govett, S. B. (1995). *School-related noise exposure in children.* Paper presented at the Association for Research in Otolaryngology Mid-Winter Meeting, St. Petersburg, FL.

Cornelisse, L., Seewald, R., & Jamieson, D. (1995). The input/output formula: A theoretical approach to the fitting of personal amplification devices. *Journal of the Acoustical Society of America, 97*(3), 1854–1864.

Erber, N. P. (1982). *Auditory training.* Washington, DC: Alexander Graham Bell Association for the Deaf.

Finitzo-Hieber, T. (1988). Classroom acoustics. In R. Roeser (Ed.), *Auditory disorders in school children* (2nd ed., pp. 221–223). New York, NY: Thieme-Stratton.

Gantz, B. J., Hansen, M. R., Turner, C. W., Oleson, J. J., Reiss, L. A., & Parkinson, A. J. (2009). Hybrid 10 clinical trial: Preliminary results. *Audiology & Neurotology, 14* (Suppl 1), 32–38.

Gstoettner W. K., van de Heyning, P., O'Connor, A. F., Morera, C., Sainz, M., Vermeire, K., et al. (2008). Electric acoustic stimulation of the auditory system: Results of a multi-centre investigation. *Acta Otolaryngologica, 128*, 968–975.

Ha, J. F., Wood, B., Krishnaswamy, J., & Rajan, G. P. (2012). Incomplete cochlear partition type II variants as an indicator of congenital partial deafness: A first report. *Otology & Neurotology, 33*, 957–962.

Jayawardena, J., Kuthubutheen, J., & Rajan, G. (2012). Hearing preservation and hearing improvement after reimplantation of pediatric and adult patients with partial deafness: A retrospective case series review. *Otology & Neurotology, 33*, 740–744.

Kuthubutheen, J., Hedne, C. N., Krishnaswamy, J., & Rajan, G. P. (2012). A case series of paediatric hearing preservation cochlear implantation: A new treatment modality for children with drug-induced or congenital partial deafness. *Audiology and Neurotology, 17*(5), 321–330.

Madell, J. M. (2010). *Pediatric amplification: Using speech perception to achieve best outcomes.* Audiologyonline e-seminar.

Moog, J. S., & Geers, A. (1990). *Early Speech Perception Test for profoundly hearing-impaired children.* St. Louis, MO: Central Institute for the Deaf.

Mueller, H. G., & Killion, M. C. (1990). An easy method for calculating the articulation index. *The Hearing Journal, 43,* 1–4.

Nober, L. W., & Nober, E. H. (1975). Auditory discrimination of learning disabled children in quiet and classroom noise. *Journal of Learning Disabilities, 8,* 656–659.

Olsen, W. O. (1998). Average speech levels and spectra in various speaking/listening conditions: A summary of the Pearson, Bennett & Fidel Report (1977). *American Journal of Audiology, 7,* 21–25.

Pearsons, K. S., Bennett, R. L., & Fidell, S. (1977). *Speech levels in various noise environments* (report no. EPA-600/1-77-025). Washington, DC: U.S. Environmental Protection Agency.

Sanders, D. (1965). Noise conditions in normal school classrooms. *Exceptional Child, 31,* 344–353.

Scollie, S., Seewald, R., Cornelisse, L., Moodie, S., Bagatto, M., Laurnagaray, D., et al. (2005). The desired sensation level multistage input/output algorithm. *Trends in Amplification, 9*(4), 159–197.

Seewald, R. C., Ross M., & Spiro, M. K. (1985). Selecting amplification characteristics for young hearing-impaired children. *Ear and Hearing, 6,* 48–51.

Skarzynski, H., & Lorens, A. (2010). Electric acoustic stimulation in children. *Advances in Otorhinolaryngology, 67,* 135–143.

Skarzynski, H., Lorens, A., D'Haese, P., Walkowiak A., Piotrowska, A., Sliwa, L., & Anderson I. (2002). Preservation of residual hearing in children and post-lingually deafened adults after cochlear implantation: An initial study. *ORL Journal of Otorhinolaryngoloy and Related Specialties, 64,* 247–253.

Skarzynski, H., Lorens, A., Piotrowska, A., & Anderson, I. (2006). Partial deafness cochlear implantation provides benefit to a new population of individuals with hearing loss. *Acta Oto-Laryngologica, 126,* 934–940.

Skinner, M. W., Holden, L. K., Holden, T. K., & Demorest, M. E. (1999). Comparison of two methods for selecting minimum stimulation levels used in programming the Nucleus 22 cochlear implant. *Journal of Speech, Language and Hearing Research, 42,* 814–828.

Skinner, M. W., Holden, L. K., Holden, T. A., Demorest, M. E., & Fourakis, M. S. (1997). Speech recognition at simulated soft, conversational, and raised-to-loud vocal efforts by adults with cochlear implants. *Journal of the Acoustical Society of America, 101*(6), 3766–3782.

Thielmeir, M. A. (1982). *Discrimination after training test.* Los Angeles, CA: House Ear Institute.

┃┃┃ 8 ┃┃┃

Role of the Speech-Language Pathologist and Teacher of the Deaf in the Postoperative Assessment of Children

Emily Lund

INTRODUCTION

Speech-language pathologists (SLP), teachers of the deaf (TOD), and in some cases, early interventionists (EI) play important roles in monitoring the progress of cochlear implant recipients. These professionals see children regularly and across various settings, and consequently, they are ideally positioned to collect data on a child's performance over time. Information about a child's progress helps a rehabilitation team to answer one key question: Is the child making the expected amount of progress as a result of his or her cochlear implant?

As in preoperative assessment, it is imperative that a team evaluating postoperative outcomes of a child (or adult) with a cochlear implant understand the principles of monitoring progress.

Additionally, professionals should understand the role of progress monitoring in future decisions that are made for a child with cochlear implants.

This chapter (a) outlines the principles of progress monitoring and recommended schedule for postoperative assessment, (b) details popular assessment and therapeutic tools used by SLPs and other educators, and (c) discusses the roles of professionals, including SLPs and TODs, in the rehabilitation process.

PRINCIPLES OF POSTOPERATIVE PROGRESS MONITORING

Progress-monitoring instruments are designed to give professionals periodic feedback about a child's skill acquisition (Francis et al., 2008). Lack of access to sound prior to implantation can cause delays across many domains, including speech, language, and academic achievement; therefore, professionals evaluating postoperative outcomes need to consider the rate at which a child with a cochlear implant is acquiring new skills. Specifically, a team must answer the following questions: What is the child's rate of progress? Has the rate of progress changed following cochlear implantation? and How does the child's progress compare to the rate expected by the cochlear implant team? Ideally, the team should answer these questions across several different domains, including speech production, language development, auditory functioning, and academic achievement.

To answer these questions, the rehabilitative team needs to agree on a regular postoperative assessment schedule. Ideally, a child who receives a cochlear implant should receive a comprehensive speech-language evaluation 6 and 12 months post-implant, and annually thereafter (see Table 8–1 for a sample schedule). In addition, professionals on the team may wish to track progress with specific measures more frequently to establish a clear rate of growth. Once a child demonstrates age-appropriate speech, language, and/or academic skills with his or her implant, the team may decide to further alter or discontinue assessment within a specific domain.

Although many assessment instruments are available to a rehabilitative team, not all of these instruments are appropriate for progress monitoring. Norm-referenced measures are designed to identify a child's delays relative to other typically developing children; they should only be administered according to a restricted schedule (e.g., only one time per year). Norm-referenced measures are not, therefore, ideal for measuring progress over a short period of time (e.g., weeks or months). Because criterion-referenced measures are designed to determine if a child has mastered a particular set of skills, some measures can be administered repeatedly over the course of a year.

Table 8–1. Sample Timeline for Postoperative Assessment

Time Post-implantation	Domains to Assess	Additional Decision Notes
6 months	Auditory skills, speech production, language skills, academic knowledge	During this period, the team will want to use only criterion-referenced measures. If progress within the first 3 months appears insufficient to the team, additional assessments within a given domain may be completed at 9 months.
12 months	Auditory skills, speech production, language skills, academic knowledge	The team may use a combination of criterion-referenced and/or norm-referenced measures to determine (a) if the child is still delayed and (b) what is his or her rate or progress.
2 years	Auditory skills, speech production, language skills, academic knowledge	If the rate of progress was slower than the rehabilitation team predicted during the first year, progress-monitoring assessments may be given every 3 months or on a similar schedule.
3 years	Auditory skills, speech production, language skills, academic knowledge	During an annual assessment, if a child demonstrates age-appropriate skills in one domain (e.g., speech production), the team may decide to discontinue testing in that domain unless a parent, therapist, or teacher raises additional concerns.
Prior to IEP (Individualized Education Plan) qualifications	Auditory skills, speech production, language skills, academic knowledge	Before a child is initially evaluated or reevaluated for an IEP, the team should complete comprehensive testing composed primarily of norm-referenced measures to determine if the child's skills are exceptional.

Professionals must monitor the progress of children with cochlear implants regularly, especially within the first year of implantation, and criterion-referenced measures provide a more effective solution than norm-referenced measures.

Many different types of criterion-referenced assessment instruments are available to professionals, including checklists, developmental scales, and progress-monitoring instruments. Checklists and developmental scales can be based on teacher report, parent report, direct observation, and/or specific items designed to elicit responses directly from a child. Progress-monitoring instruments, such as the Dynamic Indicators of Basic Early Literacy Skills assessment (DIBELS), are designed specifically for monitoring the growth of a very specific skill at set intervals (Good, Kaminski, Smith, Laimon, & Dill, 2001). The rehabilitative team may consider information from all types of instruments to estimate the rate at which a child is improving.

Progress-monitoring instruments are designed to be easy to administer, and they provide scores on a constant metric across many different test forms (Francis et al., 2008). Regular and easy administration allows a professional to take data across multiple time points without interfering with a child's typical intervention session or school day. Because the assessment instrument is administered many times, the scores a child receives should be consistent across time points. For example, if a child receives a score of 5 one week, 6 the next week, and 7 the following week, the intervals between scores of 5, 6, and 7 should indicate equal growth from the first to the second and the second to the third week.

In addition, a progress-monitoring instrument should be free from practice and form effects (Francis et al., 2008). A practice effect occurs if a child improves his or her score on an instrument because he or she is familiar with the measure, rather than because his or her skill has improved. A form effect occurs when test forms are not of equivalent difficulty. As a result, a change in a child's score may be the result of test-form difficulty, not skill improvement. For example, a test may require a child to read one paragraph one week and then a more difficult paragraph the next week. If the child has more errors in the second

paragraph, he or she is subject to a form effect, not a skill regression.

All members of a rehabilitative team should be able to evaluate the appropriateness and validity of assessments used to measure the progress of speech, language, auditory, and academic skills. In the following sections, general criterion-referenced and progress-monitoring specific instruments that are frequently used to capture change in children's development are discussed.

SPECIFIC PROGRESS-MONITORING INSTRUMENTS

Assessments of Speech Production

Popular norm-referenced measures of articulation, such as the Arizona Articulation Proficiency Scale–3 (Figure 8–1) and the Goldman-Fristoe Test of Articulation–2, were not designed to track progress over short periods of time (Fudala, 2000; Goldman & Fristoe, 2000). Consequently, SLPs must use checklists or other progress-monitoring measures to track day-to-day change in vocal development and articulation skills (Table 8–2). Some of the criterion-referenced measures discussed in Chapter 4 are appropriate for this purpose. The Rosetti Infant–Toddler Language Scale (RI-TLS) tracks early speech-sound development as a part of the expressive language subscale (Rossetti, 1990). Other clinicians may choose to use articulation inventories, such as the Central Institute for the Deaf Phonetic Inventory, which track a child's production of speech sounds in all word positions (Moog, 1989). These inventories, however, do not always provide specific ages by which a sound should be mastered, but rather provide documentation showing improvement in articulation skills over time.

Some assessments specifically designed for measuring speech-production progress are available. The Children's Speech Intelligibility Measure, for example, provides many versions of a stimulus list (Wilcox & Morris, 1999). The SLP can score a child's productions across several week-long intervals to determine if regular progress is being made. This type of instrument, however,

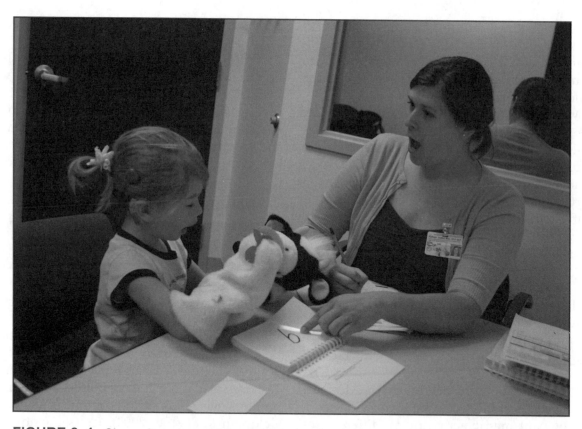

FIGURE 8–1. Shown here is an SLP administering the Arizona Articulation Proficiency Scale–3 to a 5-year-old implant recipient.

Table 8–2. Possible Measures for Progress Monitoring

Measure Name	Type of Measure	Domains Assessed	Age/ Grade Range	Information Collected
Rosetti Infant–Toddler Language Scales (RI-TLS)	Criterion referenced	Subtests: Interaction–attachment, pragmatics, gesture, play, language comprehension, language expression	0–36 months	Direct observation, behavior elicitation, parental report
Cottage Acquisition Scales for Listening, Language and Speech (CASSLS)	Criterion referenced	Forms available: pre-verbal, pre-sentence, simple sentence, complex sentence, sounds and speech	0–8 years	Direct observation, behavior elicitation, parental report
St. Gabriel's Curriculum for the Development of Audition, Language, Speech, and Cognition	Criterion referenced	Audition, speech, cognition, social interaction, fine motor skills, gross motor skills	0–6 years	Direct observation, behavior elicitation, parental report

Table 8–2. *continued*

Measure Name	Type of Measure	Domains Assessed	Age/ Grade Range	Information Collected
Central Institute for the Deaf Phonetic Inventory	Criterion referenced	Articulation	All ages	Observation
Phonetic–Phonologic Speech Evaluation Record	Criterion referenced	Articulation	All ages	Observation, behavior elicitation
Children's Speech Intelligibility Measure	Criterion referenced	Articulation	3–10 years	Behavior elicitation
MacArthur-Bates Communicative Development Inventory (CDI)	Criterion referenced	Forms: words and gestures, words and sentences	8–30 months	Direct observation, parental report
SKI-HI Language Development Scale	Criterion referenced	Receptive language, expressive language	0–5 years	Parental report
Index of Narrative Complexity	Criterion referenced	Narrative macrostructures and microstructures	School-age children	Behavior elicitation
Early Speech Perception Test (ESP)	Criterion referenced	Auditory discrimination and identification	3–12 years	Behavior elicitation
Auditory Perception Test for the Hearing Impaired, Revised (APT/HI-R)	Criterion referenced	Auditory discrimination and identification	5+ years	Behavior elicitation
Phonological Awareness Literacy Screening Measures (PALS-PreK, PALS-K, PALS-1–3)	Criterion referenced	Name writing, alphabet knowledge, beginning sound awareness, rhyme awareness, nursery rhyme knowledge, print and word awareness, letter sounds, spelling, word recognition, passage reading, comprehension, fluency	Preschool–3rd Grade	Behavior elicitation
Bracken School Readiness Assessment, Third Edition (BSRA)	Criterion referenced	Color knowledge, letter knowledge, numbers/counting, comparison/size knowledge, shape knowledge	3–6 years	Behavior elicitation
Dynamic Indicators of Basic Early Literacy Skills	Criterion referenced	Initial sound fluency, letter-naming fluency, phoneme segmentation fluency, nonsense-word fluency, oral reading fluency	Kindergarten–6th grade	Behavior elicitation

may not be appropriate for a child immediately following implantation; children develop articulation skills over the course of several years. Consequently, children may not produce age-appropriate phonemes for an extended time period following implantation. Other measures of vocal development may be used to track first-year progress.

Another widely used assessment tool, the Cottage Acquisition Scales for Listening and Spoken Language (CASSLS), allows parents and therapists to compare listening, language, speech, and cognitive skill development to a timeline; a child's listening age is compared with his or her skill acquisition across those domains (Wilkes, 1999). The test forms for this measure are divided into preverbal, presentence, simple sentence, and complex-sentences levels, and one additional form is available to measure speech-sound production. SLPs, TODs, or EIs can use these forms to compare a child's skills in one domain (e.g., receptive language) with another (e.g., speech production). Other scales and checklists, including those from St. Gabriel's Curriculum for the Development of Audition, Language, Speech, and Cognition, the Phonetic–Phonologic Speech Evaluation Record: A Manual, can also provide useful benchmarks for professionals to use to gauge children's progress (Tuohy, Brown, & Mercer-Moseley, 2005; Ling, 1991). If a child is not developing speech-production skills at the rate anticipated by the cochlear implant team, the group may discuss altering a child's cochlear implant settings or changing intervention techniques.

Assessments of Language

As with speech production, many common language tests, such as the Preschool Language Scale–5, Peabody Picture Vocabulary Test–4, or the Clinical Evaluation of Language Fundamentals–4, are not designed or appropriate for capturing change in specific language skills across short periods of time (Zimmerman, Steiner, & Pond, 2010; Dunn & Dunn, 2006; Semel, Wiig, & Secord, 2003). A rehabilitation team may instead turn to criterion-referenced measures designed to capture change in a child's ability to produce language

structures (e.g., acquisition of the past-tense grammatical morpheme "ed"). A child's needs identified during baseline testing should determine which measures are appropriate for tracking the progress of language skills.

Language-skill progress-monitoring instruments have been recently developed for children who have sufficient language to complete a language sample. For example, the Index of Narrative Complexity provides a scale for rating the quality of narrative productions over time (Petersen, Gillam, & Gillam, 2008); however, these types of measures are not necessarily appropriate for a recently implanted child, and they should only be used with older children who have either had an implant for many years or have acquired an implant due to a progressive loss.

Criterion-based measures and checklists of language skills designed for children with cochlear implants are available. The aforementioned criterion-referenced measures, such as the RI-TLS, the CASLLS, St. Gabriel's Curriculum for the Development of Audition, Language, Speech, and Cognition, SKI-HI Developmental Language Scale, and the MacArthur-Bates Communicative Development Inventories (see Chapter 4), can all be used to track early language development in children (Rossetti, 1990; Wilkes, 1999; Tuohy et al., 2005; Watkins, 1979; Fenson et al., 2006). These scales can capture changes in language performance during the first year of implant use.

Assessments of Auditory Skills

Auditory skills are among the skills most likely to improve quickly post-implantation (Robbins, Koch, Osberger, Zimmerman-Phillips, & Kishon-Rabin, 2004). A child's early auditory skills may change his or her development across other domains; therefore, capturing change in skills directly related to auditory function is one of the most important tasks for a child's rehabilitative team. The Early Speech Perception Test (ESP) and the Auditory Perception Test for the Hearing Impaired (APT/HI-R), described in Chapter 4, can be used for the purposes of progress monitoring (Moog & Geers, 1990; Allen & Serwatka, 2008); however, neither test can be administered very quickly. Consequently, other measures of auditory development may be more useful for frequent tracking of changes in auditory development.

Many curricula and checklists allow professionals to track a child's auditory development. St. Gabriel's Curriculum for the Development of Audition, Language, Speech, and Cognition as well as the Cottage Acquisition Scales for Listening, Language, and Speech provide scales specific to auditory development (Wilkes, 1999; Tuohy et al., 2005). The Functional Auditory Performance Indicators Scale (FAPI) also assesses auditory development across the following categories: sound awareness, meaningful sound, auditory feedback, localization, auditory discrimination, short-term memory, and linguistic auditory processing (Stredler-Brown & Johnson, 2004). Professionals, in collaboration with parents, can use these various scales to generate a profile describing a child's listening skills and progress over short periods of time. If a child is not acquiring early auditory skills, the team may choose to adjust his or her implant settings to ensure maximal benefit from the device.

Assessments of Academic Knowledge

A variety of instruments are available for tracking progress in academic skill sets, including phonological awareness, reading, writing, and mathematical skill development. TODs, and in some cases, SLPs, can regularly administer these instruments to describe a child's academic progress post-implantation.

Many classroom curricula provide assessment tools to track a child's knowledge of recently taught concepts. Other published tools track progress across broader sets of skills. The Dynamic Indicators of Basic Early Literacy Skills (DIBELS), for example, measures growth in skills related to reading (Good et al., 2001). Other tools, including the Phonological Awareness Literacy Screening (PALS) or the Bracken School Readiness Assessment (third edition), can also be used periodically to measure a child's skill mastery (Invernizzi, Meier, Swank, & Juel, 2004; Bracken, 2007). TODs can collaborate with general education teachers to determine whether a child's rate of academic

skill progress is appropriate for his or her listening experience. In addition, the TOD can observe the ways in which a child's speech and language skills impact his or her academic achievement. If a child's academic progress is inconsistent with his or her progress across other domains, the team may choose to provide additional educational support to a child in his or her school setting.

THERAPY POST-IMPLANTATION

After a child receives a cochlear implant and gains access to sound, possibly for the first time, parents often need guidance not only to use the implant equipment, but also to learn to use the most appropriate and efficient language-facilitation techniques. SLPs, TODs, and EIs all can play a role in helping a parent or teacher develop the tools needed to promote language development. To work effectively as a team, all team members must (a) understand a child's current level of functioning, (b) recognize the next stage of development (goal of intervention), (c) know the best techniques for encouraging development, and (d) agree what behaviors will provide the evidence that a goal is met. Establishing these guidelines within team meetings ensures that families and professionals are able to work together toward a common goal.

The parent's role is central to developing and achieving intervention goals. All families must fit intervention for their child into their daily routines; thus, professionals should be sensitive to the needs and capabilities of a family when planning treatment. It is not the professional's sole responsibility to determine goals and how they will be met; rather, professionals bring knowledge of typical and atypical development, as well as intervention techniques to the family, who can then make decisions about goals and treatment with guidance. One effective way of assessing a family's strengths and needs is to conduct a routines-based interview (McWilliam, Casey, & Sims, 2009). A routines-based interview requires interventionists to ask in-depth questions about a family's typical day to evaluate opportunities for communicative interventions.

SLPs, TODs, and EIs can help a family enhance their child's development by teaching a family about a child's expected trajectory of development. A clear understanding of the stages a child may progress through will help a rehabilitation team to develop treatment goals and methods.

The following sections review the possible stages of postoperative development and implications for intervention. This model assumes that a child has not previously had access to sound and is beginning the language-learning process with no knowledge of language. For children who may have a progressive or acquired loss, these principles can still be applied at appropriate stages (i.e., if a child already has sound detection, therapists can look to the next stage of development to set their goals and expectations).

Therapy Immediately Following Implantation

Many parents (and even professionals) are often disappointed to learn that most children are not prepared to listen, respond, and speak immediately following activation of a cochlear implant. In the same way that babies receive a year of language input before producing their first words, children with cochlear implants need time to develop their auditory skills prior to producing speech. Despite a lack of speech, children in the early stages of auditory development should make observable gains that professionals can monitor and encourage.

Throughout a child's first months postimplantation, the people who spend the most time with a child throughout his or her day (e.g., parents, babysitters, teachers) play a vital role in helping a child develop these auditory skills. Early intervention, therefore, should focus on teaching caretakers to use effective strategies throughout the day. The role of the professional, in this case, is as a parent coach rather than teacher to the child.

According to Erber's four-level model of auditory development, the first step in auditory-skill acquisition is developing sound-detection skills (i.e., determining if a sound is present or absent) (Erber, 1982). Because many children are not used to attending to information coming from an auditory channel, children with cochlear implants have to learn to detect and attend to different types of environmental sounds. Basic detection abilities often develop quickly (Niparko, 2000). Within a day of initial implant activation, a child may begin to respond to sounds presented in the absence of other distractions; however, differentiated responses to different environmental sounds may develop more slowly over the first couple of months of sound access (Moore & Shannon, 2009). To encourage sound detection, the rehabilitation team will want to draw a child's attention to sounds of different types. These sounds can include staccato, novel sounds that occur in the environment (e.g., the telephone ringing, the doorbell ringing, the microwave beeping) and continuous, "white-noise" sounds (e.g., the dishwasher running). Sounds present in the environment of any child vary, so environmental sound-based activities are often unique to a specific family.

Following the development of auditory detection, children should begin to discriminate between different sounds, and to associate words with their referents (Erber, 1982). A child who is just learning to listen is not necessarily prepared to discriminate between individual phonemes of words (e.g., "map" versus "mat") (Niparko, 2000). Prior to developing those skills, children with cochlear implants first learn to discriminate between suprasegmental features of speech. Suprasegmental features include the pitch (high or low), loudness (loud or soft), and duration (long or short) of groups of speech sounds; thus, a child who is unable to distinguish between two words of similar duration with different phonemes (e.g., "cat" versus "dog") may be able to distinguish between words of varying gross duration ("ice cream cone" versus "cat"). Children vary in their recognition of suprasegmental differences between words: some children develop this ability early, whereas others take up to many months post-implant to discriminate between sounds (Snow & Ertmer, 2012). A rehabilitation team can emphasize the development of discrimination abilities while encouraging a child to connect sounds to objects. For example, the parent, SLP, TOD, and EI may choose to label objects in a child's environment with sounds that have different suprasegmental properties (e.g., teaching the child that the cat says "meeeooww" and the dog says "woof woof"). Noting a child's ability to discriminate between and comprehend those labels provides a team with information about a child's auditory development. Acoustically highlighting features of speech may improve a child's early ability to learn and even use words (Simser & Estabrooks, 2001).

In addition to learning to discriminate word-level differences, within the first 8 months of listening children with cochlear implants may also learn to recognize rote phrases (Robbins, 2005). These phrases include those used frequently in everyday life, such as "shut the door," "sit down," "let's go!" etc. The rote phrases that an individual child hears likely vary across families. Parents and professionals can encourage the development of rote-phrase recognition by highlighting consistent phrases during a child's daily routines (see Table 8–3). Furthermore, parents and professionals can track children's responses to these phrases when presented through audition alone (without visual cues). If a child is able to anticipate an action (e.g., looking to the door) following an auditory-only presentation of a rote phrase (e.g., "let's go!"), he or she is showing signs of rote phrase comprehension.

During the initial months following a child's implantation, parents should begin to use techniques for making certain sounds, words, and phrases acoustically salient to children (Simser & Estabrooks, 2001). These techniques, often labeled "acoustic highlighting," may contribute to children's ability to develop discrimination abilities. Parents can use many different acoustic-highlighting strategies within the context of their daily lives (see Table 8–3). For example, placing key words at the end of a phrase, slowing the rate of speech, or increasing the amplitude of a specific word improves the acoustic salience of that word to a child with hearing loss. The rehabilitation team can work together to ensure that a child's attention is drawn to acoustically salient sounds, words, and phrases during the first months of implant use.

Even before children with cochlear implants begin using words to communicate, they can learn about the conventional use of spoken language (Goldin-Meadow & Mylander, 1984). Professional- and parent-led intervention activities can help

Table 8–3. Acoustic Highlighting Strategies

Strategy	Example
Limit background noise.	Turn off the television, dishwasher, or air conditioner when interacting with the child.
Speak near the cochlear implant microphone.	
Provide repetitions of key information.	Instead of giving a direction one time, provide multiple opportunities for a child to grasp the message (e.g., "Look, the shoes are *red*! I see *red* shoes! They're *red*!").
Limit the length of spoken instruction.	Instead of giving two to three instructions at one time, divide the key points into several parts (e.g., "Go get your coat . . . and go to the door.").
Slow the rate of speech.	
Place key words at the end of an utterance.	Give key semantic information at the end of the sentence (e.g., "Go to the *door*.").

children to understand that words are meaningful, that words can control the actions of others, and that people converse using sequences of speech sounds. Activities that encourage understanding of these communicative principles are often the same types of activities children participate in as infants, such as imitating nonsense sounds and syllables. Although these activities may not seem appropriate for children beyond infancy, parents and professionals should target these early-developing skills with newly implanted children who have little to no spoken language.

Therapy During the Early Stages of Language Learning

As children develop the ability to discriminate phonemes, they begin to understand and use words (Erber, 1982). Professionals can use published materials to track changes in a child's ability to discriminate between increasingly similar words. For example, the SPICE curriculum provides both auditory-training activities and progress-tracking scales designed to capture a child's ability to differentiate between minimally different words (Moog, Biedenstein, & Davidson, 1995). Although research does not currently prove or disprove that behavioral therapy can increase or decrease a child's discrimination abilities, professionals can track this development to set appropriate corresponding language goals.

Once a child is able to perceive and identify individual words, he or she can develop word-learning skills. To acquire new vocabulary, children with hearing loss benefit from frequent repetition (Simser & Estabrooks, 2001). Professionals may want to focus intervention on commonly used words and phrases during this phase of development to ensure that children are repeatedly hearing target vocabulary words throughout the day. This initial focus on frequently occurring, functional vocabulary words may provide children with the ability to interact with others during routines (e.g., mealtime or playtime).

As children learn and begin to combine words, they may develop knowledge of basic syntax and morphology. Children in the early stages of language learning often use sentence frames to com-

municate. Sentence frames are frequently used phrases that can be combined with other words to communicate a message. For example, "where's the _____" and "look at _____" are sentence frames often used in child-directed speech (Cameron-Faulkner, Lieven, & Tomasello, 2003). Parents and professionals can encourage children with cochlear implants to use sentence frames and longer sentence structures by recasting and expanding sentences (DesJardin & Eisenberg, 2007). For example, a child might say, "look at dog," and a parent could recast and expand the utterance by replying, "Yes! Look at that big dog in the park!" During this phase of development, children also begin to use grammatical morphemes. Many morphemes in the English language are marked by high frequency, unstressed phonemes (e.g., plural "s" and regular past-tense "-ed"). These particular morphemes can be especially difficult for children with hearing loss to perceive and, consequently, produce (Spencer, Tye-Murray, & Tomblin, 1998). SLPs and TODs can help parents to recognize these morphemes in connected speech and highlight or emphasize them for their child with a cochlear implant. Both parents and professionals should continue to use acoustic highlighting techniques (see Table 8–3) during this stage of development to ensure that a child has access to important linguistic information.

Preschool children with cochlear implants, in addition to developing basic linguistic knowledge, can begin to acquire early literacy skills. For example, children may begin to develop early print knowledge and phonological awareness. Print knowledge may include concepts of print (e.g., reading books from left to right) and word knowledge (e.g., words are comprised of letters, letters represent sounds). Phonological awareness refers to the ability to recognize and analyze the sounds of words separate from their meaning. Children can acquire both print knowledge and phonological awareness through shared storybook reading (Desjardin, Ambrose, & Eisenberg, 2009). SLPs and TODs may focus intervention on mothers' use of facilitative techniques. Throughout the early stages of language and literacy development, parents and professionals can work as partners to ensure that language-learning opportunities are maximized throughout a child's day.

Therapy During Later Stages of Language Learning

Children with cochlear implants may develop language skills rapidly in the first 2 to 3 years post-implantation (Nicholas & Geers, 2007). Despite growth during this period, however, it is likely that a child's language skills will continue to lag behind those of peers with normal hearing; thus, professionals play a role in continuing to help a child with cochlear implants to acquire the necessary speech and language skills to function academically and socially.

Children with cochlear implants vary greatly in their auditory working memory skills and in their ability to listen in unaccommodating environments (Dowell, Dettman, Blamey, Barker, & Clark, 2002). Professionals can work to increase a child's confidence listening to sentences of increasing length and in noisy environments, and to make accommodations in the child's classroom and home environment to provide optimal listening experiences. Both parents and professionals can engage a child in activities that require him or her to follow directions of increasing complexity (e.g., "Get the red crayon and put it in the box on the shelf"). Experience listening to complicated directions may build a child's confidence in his or her ability to retain and comprehend this type of information in real-world settings (Cole & Flexer, 2007). Similarly, parents and professionals can give a child experience listening through noisy environments. In addition, SLPs and TODs can work with general educators and parents to examine the listening demands placed on a child in his or her natural environment. When a child is asked to learn and retain new academic information, ideally he or she should have the opportunity to learn without interference from noise (Schafer & Thibodeau, 2006). Reduction of background noise can improve a child's learning experience.

SLPs may also want to devote some individual therapy time to correcting a child's lingering speech-production errors. After a child is able to perceive and discriminate individual speech phonemes, he or she can begin to correct them in conversational speech; however, some children with cochlear implants need intervention to overcome poor speech-production habits (Tobey, Geers, Sun-darrajan, & Shin, 2011). Parents and professionals can help a child to monitor his or her own speech production throughout the day to identify and correct errors.

Even after a child with cochlear implants has mastered basic grammar skills, he or she may still have subtle language deficits. Children with hearing loss, including children with cochlear implants, have less robust lexical knowledge than children with normal hearing. Vocabulary deficits can impact a child's ability to complete academic work. For example, a child with hearing loss may struggle with a social studies assignment if he or she does not understand most of the vocabulary used. Preteaching vocabulary and language structures unfamiliar to a child can improve his or her ability to function in a general education classroom setting (Stith & Drasgow, 2005). Children with hearing loss may also struggle to understand nonliteral language (e.g., idioms, sarcasm) (Schorr, Roth, & Fox, 2008). SLPs, TODs, and parents can all work to explicitly teach a child about nonliteral uses of language. A child's individual language deficits should drive the goals of his or her therapy.

As children with cochlear implants enter elementary school, rehabilitative teams should monitor the acquisition of literacy-related skills. Children with hearing loss, including children with cochlear implants, generally have poor reading outcomes related to both decoding and comprehension (Geers & Hayes, 2011). Children with skill deficits related to either decoding or comprehension may need supplemental instruction in those areas. SLPs in particular can apply their specialized knowledge of phonological awareness to a rehabilitative team's intervention plan (Spencer, Schuele, Guillot, & Lee, 2008).

Adult Intervention

In addition to serving children with cochlear implants, SLPs and TODs can play a role in the rehabilitation of adults who receive cochlear implants. By the time an adult receives an implant, it is likely that he or she has already had the linguistic and academic training necessary for him or her to function in the world. A cochlear implant, however, provides an adult with new levels of access to sound. As a result, adults with cochlear implants may be able to develop better auditory-functioning skills or speech skills post-implant (Fu, Galvin, Wang, & Nogaki, 2005).

A professional can guide an adult with a cochlear implant through structured exercises to improve his or her listening skills over the course of the first year post-implantation (Caposecco, Hickson, & Pedley, 2011). Adults, like children, can move through several stages of auditory functioning. First, an adult may begin with simple detection exercises (e.g., is the sound there or not?), move into discrimination exercises (e.g., differentiate sounds and words of varying length, pitch, loudness, and phonemes), and then to comprehension of longer phrases. The amount of gain an adult can make may be limited depending on his or her pre-implant language skills and duration of deafness (Caposecco et al., 2011). SLPs or TODs may provide structured guidance to an adult to help him or her reach maximum listening potential.

Improved access to sound also may provide some adults with an opportunity to change articulation habits. Instructing adults in new articulation patterns can be similar to working with a school-age child. An SLP can talk directly to the adult about the correct physiologic way to produce a phoneme and provide opportunities for production across words, phrases, and sentences in initial, medial, and final positions. The amount of change an adult is able to make is likely dependent on his or her speech-perception ability and willingness to change habits.

CONCLUSION

Rehabilitative teams, which may include parents, audiologists, TODs, SLPs, EIs, and many other professionals, must work together to evaluate a child's postoperative outcomes. Progress monitoring informs decisions about intervention. To communicate about progress and intervention, all members of a rehabilitative team should meet regularly. If the progress-monitoring and inter-vention expectations of various team members are clear from the beginning of treatment, all parties can contribute to a child's progress. Using the various progress-monitoring tools available, rehabilitative teams can track a child's growth to maximize his or her spoken-language outcomes.

REFERENCES

Allen, S. G., & Serwatka, T. S. (2008). *Auditory perception test for the hearing impaired* (Rev. ed.). San Diego, CA: Plural.

Bracken, B. A. (2007). *Bracken school readiness assessment* (3rd ed.). San Antonio, TX: The Psychological Corporation.

Cameron-Faulkner, T., Lieven, E., & Tomasello, M. (2003). A construction based analysis of child directed speech. *Cognitive Science, 27,* 843–873.

Caposecco, A., Hickson, L., & Pedley, K. (2011). Cochlear implant outcomes in adults and adolescents with early-onset hearing loss. *Ear and Hearing, 33,* 209–220.

Cole, E. B., & Flexer, C. A. (2007). *Children with hearing loss: Developing listening and talking birth to six.* San Diego, CA: Plural.

Desjardin, J., Ambrose, S., & Eisenberg, L. (2009). Literacy skills in children with cochlear implants: The importance of early oral language and joint storybook reading. *Journal of Deaf Studies and Deaf Education, 14*(1), 22–43.

DesJardin, J. L., & Eisenberg, L. S. (2007). Maternal contributions: Supporting language development in young children with cochlear implants. *Ear and Hearing, 28l,* 456–469.

Dowell, R. C., Dettman, S. J., Blamey, P. J., Barker, E. J., & Clark, G. M. (2002). Speech perception in children using cochlear implants: Prediction of long term outcomes. *Cochlear Implants International, 3,* 1–18.

Dunn, L. A., & Dunn, L. M. (2006). *Peabody Picture Vocabulary Test* (PPVT-4) (4th ed.). Circle Pines, MN: AGS.

Erber, N. (1982). *Auditory training.* Washington, D. C.: Alexander Graham Bell Association for the Deaf.

Fenson, L., Marchman, V., Thal, D., Dale, P., Reznick, S., & Bates, E. (2006). *The MacArthur communicative development inventories: User's guide and technical manual* (2nd ed.). Baltimore, MD: Brookes.

Francis, D. J., Sanit, K. L., Barr, C., Fletcher, J. M., Varisco, A., & Foorman, B. R. (2008). Form effects on the estimation of students' oral reading fluency using DIBELS. *Journal of School Psychology, 46,* 315–342.

Fu, Q. J., Galvin, J., Wang, X., & Nogaki, G. (2005). Moderate auditory training can improve speech production of adult cochlear implant patients. *Acoustics Research Letters Online, 3,* 106–111.

Fudala, J. B. (2000). *Arizona articulation proficiency scale (AAPS-3)* (3rd rev. ed.). Los Angeles, CA: Western Psychological Services.

Geers, A. E., & Hayes, H. (2011). Reading, writing, and phonological processing skills of adolescents with 10 or more years of cochlear implant experience. *Ear and Hearing, 32,* 49–59.

Goldin-Meadow, S., & Mylander, C. (1984). Gestural communication in deaf children: The effects and non-effects of parental input on early language development. *Monographs of the Society for Research in Child Development, 49,* 1–151.

Goldman, R., & Fristoe, M. (2000). *Goldman Fristoe test of articulation (GFTA-2)* (2nd ed.). Circle Pines, MN: AGS.

Good, R. H., Kaminski, R. A., Smith, S., Laimon, D., & Dill, S. (2001). *Dynamic indicators of basic early literacy skills (DIBELS)* (5th ed.). Eugene, OR: University of Oregon.

Invernizzi, M., Meier, J. D., Swank, L., & Juel, C. (2004). *PALS: Phonological awareness literacy screening.* Charlottesville, VA: University of Virginia Press.

Ling, D. (1991). *Phonetic–phonologic speech evaluation record: A manual.* Washington, DC: Alexander Graham Bell Association for the Deaf.

McWilliam, R. A., Casey, A. M., & Sims, J. (2009). The routines-based interview: A method for gathering information and assessing needs. *Infant & Young Children, 22,* 224–233.

Moog, J. S. (1989). *Central Institute for the Deaf phonetic inventory.* St. Louis, MO: Central Institute for the Deaf.

Moog, J., Biedenstein, J., & Davidson, L. (1995). *SPICE: the Speech Perception Instructional Curriculum and Evaluation.* St. Louis, MO: Central Institute for the Deaf.

Moog, J. S., & Geers, A. (1990). *Early Speech Perception Test for profoundly hearing-impaired children.* St. Louis, MO: Central Institute for the Deaf.

Moore, D. R., & Shannon, R. V. (2009). Beyond cochlear implants: Awakening the deafened brain. *Nature Neuroscience, 12,* 686–691.

Nicholas, J. G., & Geers, A. E. (2007). Will they catch up? The role of age at cochlear implantation in the spoken language development of children with profound hearing loss. *Journal of Speech, Language and Hearing Research, 50,* 1048–1062.

Niparko, J. (2000). *Cochlear implants principles and practices* (2nd ed.). Baltimore, MD: Lippincott, Williams and Wilkins.

Petersen, D. B., Gillam, S. L., & Gillam, R. B. (2008). Emerging procedures in narrative assessment: The index of narrative complexity. *Topics in Language Disorders, 28,* 115–130.

Robbins, A. M. (2005). *Clinical Red Flags for slow progress in children with cochlear implants. Loud and clear.* Valencia, CA: Advanced Bionics.

Robbins, A. M., Koch, D. B., Osberger, M. J., Zimmerman-Phillips, S., & Kishon-Rabin, L. (2004). Effect of age at cochlear implantation on auditory skill development in infants and toddlers. *Archives of Otolaryngology—Head & Neck Surgery, 130,* 570–574.

Rossetti, L. (1990). *Rosetti Infant–Toddler Language Scale (RI-TLS).* East Moline, IL: LinguiSystems.

Semel, E., Wiig, E. H., & Secord, W. A. (2003). *Clinical Evaluation of Language Fundamentals (CELF-4)* (4th ed.). San Antonio, TX: The Psychological Corporation.

Schafer, E. C., & Thibodeau, L. M. (2006). Speech recognition in noise in children with cochlear implants while listening in bilateral, bimodal, and FM-system arrangements. *American Journal of Audiology, 15,* 114–126.

Schorr, E. A., Roth, F. P., & Fox N. A. A. (2008). Comparison of the speech and language skills of children with cochlear implants and children with normal hearing. *Communicable Disease Quarterly, 29,* 195–210.

Simser, J., & Estabrooks, W. (2001). What is the hand cue? What is acoustic highlighting? In W. Estabrooks (Ed.), *50 frequently asked questions about auditory verbal therapy.* Toronto, Canada: Learning to Listen Foundation.

Snow, D. P., & Ertmer, D. J. (2012). Children's development of intonation during the first year of cochlear implant experience. *Clinical Linguistics and Phonetics, 26,* 51–70.

Spencer, E. J., Schuele, C. M., Guillot, K. M., & Lee, M. W. (2008). Phonemic awareness skill of speech-language pathologists and other educators. *Language, Speech, and Hearing Services in Schools, 39,* 512–520.

Spencer, L., Tye-Murray, N., & Tomblin, J. B. (1998). The production of English inflectional morphology, speech production and listening performance in children with cochlear implants. *Ear and Hearing, 19,* 310–318.

Stith, J., & Drasgow, E. (2005). Including children with cochlear implants in regular education classrooms. *Teaching Exceptional Children Plus, 2,* 1–9.

Stredler-Brown, A., & Johnson, C. D. (2004). *Functional auditory performance indicators: An integrated approach to auditory skill development (FAPI)*. Denver, CO: Colorado Department of Special Education.

Tobey, E. A., Geers, A. E., Sundarrajan, M., & Shin, S. (2011). Factors influencing speech production in elementary and school-aged cochlear implant users. *Ear and Hearing, 32*, 27–38.

Tuohy, J., Brown, J., & Mercer-Moseley, C. (2005). *St. Gabriel's curriculum for the development of audition, language, speech, cognition, early communication, social interaction, fine motor skills, and gross motor skills* (2nd ed.). Sydney, Australia: St. Gabriel's Auditory-Verbal Early Intervention Centre.

Watkins, S. (1979). *SKI-HI Language Development Scale.* Logan, UT: SKI-HI Institute.

Wilcox, K., & Morris, S. (1999). *Children's Speech Intelligibility Measure.* London, UK: The Psychological Corporation.

Wilkes, E. M. (1999). *Cottage Acquisition Scales for Listening, Language, and Speech.* San Antonio, TX: Sunshine Cottage School for Deaf Children.

Zimmerman, I. L., Steiner, B. S., & Pond, R. E. (2010). *Preschool Language Scale (PLS-5)* (5th ed.). San Antonio, TX: The Psychological Corporation.

9

Assessing Pre- and Postoperative Outcomes for Adults and Children: What Does the Future Hold and What Might We Be Missing?

René H. Gifford

INTRODUCTION

This primary purpose of this text is to provide a handbook for clinicians who assess pre- and post-implant performance and overall outcomes for cochlear implant recipients. The focus is on current best practices and considerations for patient management in our current clinical environment. A recurring theme is that cochlear implants and patient management have both evolved rapidly since the FDA approved multichannel implants for adults and children in 1985 and 1990, respectively. Given this evolution, it follows that an expected element of our future is that clinical practices and patient management will most certainly change. It is also likely that we are missing critical elements that are relevant to a patient's candidacy and post-operative assessment—even today.

This chapter discusses the components of cochlear implant candidacy and postoperative assessment that we may be overlooking such as risk for cognitive decline, listening effort, auditory-related fatigue, and multisensory assessment. As with assessing candidacy for cochlear implantation, these metrics may ultimately also prove useful for determining candidacy for a second cochlear implant, a decision that is not currently validated via clear-cut, clinical criterion.

RISK FOR COGNITIVE DECLINE

Dementia and Link with Hearing Loss

According to the 2002 World Assembly on Aging report (United Nations, 2002), over the next 50 years, the global life expectancy at age 60 years will increase by over 22 years representing an 18% gain since 2000 to 2005. The projected gains in life expectancy are even greater for individuals living to older ages. At 80 years, life expectancy is expected to increase by almost 10 years (a 22% gain over estimates from 2000 to 2005). The 2011 Global Health and Aging report (World Health Organization, 2011) states that we are entering an era in which the number of individuals over 65 years outweighs the number children under age 5 years; thus, it is not just a global increase in life expectancy—we are observing the aging of the world's population. Figure 9–1 shows the shift in the percentage of older versus younger persons from 1950 and projected to 2050. Such a rapid shift in the world's aged population brings with it a number of societal, economic, and health-related issues.

One of the health-related consequences of an aging population is a greater incidence of dementia. The incidence of dementia increases dramatically with age every decade over age 60 years. Multiple reports have estimated that the overall prevalence of dementia is expected to double over the next 20 years, reaching a global prevalence of 1 in 85 individuals *of all ages* by the year 2050 (Ferri et al., 2005; Prince & Jackson, 2009). Alzheimer's Disease International (Prince & Jackson, 2009) reports that in North America, over 30% of individuals age 85 years and older, and nearly 40% of those over 90 years, have dementia; thus, it is a reality that clinicians working with the adult pop-

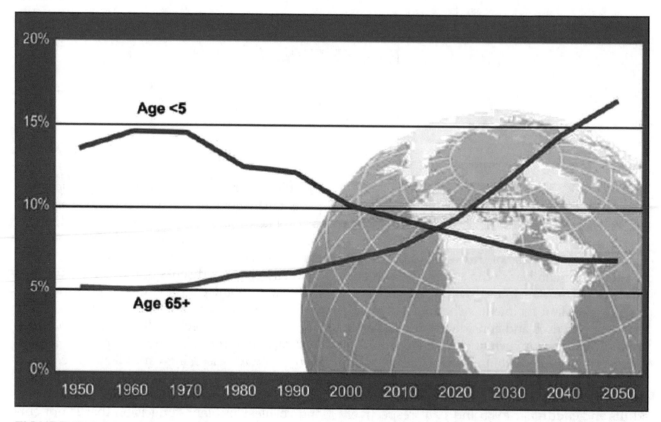

FIGURE 9–1. The shift in the percentage of older versus younger persons from 1950 and projected to 2050 is shown. (From United Nations, 2011).

ulation will be encountering individuals exhibiting signs of cognitive decline.

As of 2008, it was estimated that 34.3 million Americans (i.e., over 10% of the U.S. population) had significant hearing loss (Kochkin, 2008; U.S. Census, 2010). There are a number of recent reports demonstrating a link between age-related hearing loss (presbycusis) and dementia. Presbycusis is related to poorer cognitive functioning (Lin et al., 2011a; Tay et al., 2006) and incident dementia (Lin, Niparko, & Ferrucci, 2011b) as compared with age-matched individuals with normal or near-normal hearing. Lin (2012) reported that older adults with even mild hearing loss have a twofold risk of incident dementia. Older individuals with severe-to-profound hearing loss have a fivefold increased risk of developing dementia. This is the population of individuals that will most generally be seen in the cochlear implant clinic.

The underlying mechanisms for the association between presbycusis and dementia are not fully understood. Lin (2012) explained that there are many possible mechanisms including the effects of hearing loss on cortical processing (Peelle, Troiani, Grossman, & Wingfield, 2011), increasing cognitive load (Wingfield, Tun, & McCoy, 2005), as well as social isolation. Might it be the case that mitigating the communicative and social isolation effects of severe hearing loss with cochlear implantation may also decrease the risk of developing dementia? Current research does not allow us to definitively answer this question at this point in time. Future research on this topic, if confirmatory, could translate to further expansion in criteria for adult cochlear implantation.

Primary care physicians are acutely aware of the need for early identification of cognitive decline in order to implement an effective treatment plan (e.g., Simmons, Hartmann, & Dejoseph, 2011; Galvin & Sadowsky, 2012; Moran et al., 2012). For older individuals with significant hearing loss *and* cognitive decline, it may be the case that early and aggressive audiologic/otologic management may ultimately play a substantial role in the overall treatment for the individual. This could also mean that clinical audiologists may one day play a role in the *screening* for cognitive impairment in our adult patient population. Such a widespread screening may also provide the cochlear implant team with important information about which patients should be referred for neuropsychology or neurology consultation—a referral that might not be made unless an individual is seen regularly by his or her primary care physician and exhibits signs of cognitive decline during examination.

There are a number of available screening instruments for cognitive impairment. One of the most widely used tools is the Mini-Mental State Examination (MMSE) (Folstein, Folstein, & McHugh, 1975). The MMSE is a validated screening tool of cognitive function and administration takes approximately 5 to 10 min. The MMSE includes tests of orientation, attention, memory, language, and visuospatial skills. Table 9–1 provides an example question from the MMSE for each of the subscales.

Table 9–1. Example Questions Gauging Each of the Five Subscales for the Mini-Mental State Examination (*MMSE*)

MMSE Subscale	Example Question
Orientation	What is today's date?
Attention	Count backward from 100 by sevens.
Memory	Recall items identified earlier in the assessment.
Language	Construct a sentence about anything.
Visuospatial skills	Patient is shown a picture of two intersecting polygons and is asked to copy the picture.

Points are scored for every portion of a question answered correctly with a maximum of 30 possible points. Generally a score of 25 to 30 represents normal cognition with scores 24 and lower representing some degree of cognitive decline.

Another commonly used, validated screening tool for cognitive impairment is the **Mo**ntreal **C**ognitive **A**ssessment (MoCA) test (Nasreddine et al., 2005). The appeal of the MoCA is its ease of use, time required for administration (<10 minutes), and its sensitivity to mild forms of cognitive decline that may be missed on other screening instruments (e.g., Nazem et al., 2009; Freitas et al., 2011; Larner, 2012). The MoCA can be administered visually—without auditory cues—which is critical for the preoperative administration during cochlear implant evaluation. The MoCA assesses eight cognitive domains including attention and concentration, executive function, memory, language, visuoconstruction, conceptual thinking, mathematical calculation, and orientation. The maximum total score for all items is 30 points and just as with the MMSE, a score of 25 or lower indicates cognitive impairment.

There have been recent reports of cochlear implant programs including some type of cognitive assessment in the candidacy evaluation (Rossi-Katz & Arehart, 2011). A report by Heydebrand, Hale, Potts, and Skinner (2007), however, found no correlation between preoperative measures of general cognitive function and postoperative speech-understanding outcomes for 37 adult implant recipients ranging in age from 23 to 80 years. The obvious limitations of the study were a small sample size and a broad range of participants' ages with many participants not likely to be at risk for cognitive impairment; thus, a larger-scale assessment of the relationship between preoperative cognitive function and postoperative outcomes is needed.

On other measures of cognitive function, including general intelligence and working memory, there have been reports of a correlation with postoperative speech understanding for both adults (Lyxell et al., 1996; Heydebrand et al., 2007) and children (Pisoni, 2000; Steven et al., 2011). Most cochlear implant programs do not routinely assess cognitive status of pediatric implant candidates, with the exception of older children who

may exhibit signs of global developmental delay. The primary reason is that many children with significant hearing loss, in the absence of obvious comorbidities such as cerebral palsy and Down syndrome, are implanted at such young ages that signs of impaired cognition may not yet be evident.

LISTENING EFFORT AND FATIGUE

Hearing loss is known to increase the effort expended for cognitive and linguistic processes (e.g., Pichora-Fuller, 2007; Zekveld et al., 2007; Ronnberg et al., 2008; Shinn-Cunningham & Best, 2008; Kramer, Zekveld, & Houtgast, 2009; Hetu, Riverin, Lalande, Getty, & St-Cyr, 1988; Nachtegaal et al., 2009). This has also been referred to as *listening effort*, which specifically refers to the resources expended for attention and cognition that are required for speech understanding (e.g., Downs, 1982; Feuerstein, 1992; Hicks & Tharpe, 2002; Fraser, Gagne, Alepins, & Dubois, 2010; Gosselin & Gagne, 2011). This is not unexpected as individuals with hearing loss, particularly those with demanding professional and/or social listening environments, report that by the end of the day they experience substantial fatigue. An obvious question is: Should we be including estimates of expended listening effort in our test battery for cochlear implant candidate selection? Although an individual is able to achieve above-criterion-level performance on a sentence-recognition metric does not mean that he or she did not experience significant difficulty with the task. Perhaps another way to phrase the question is: Should individuals who happen to be better at top-down processing (i.e., filling in the gaps) be penalized by withholding cochlear implant candidacy despite having significant communicative difficulty?

Physiologic Biomarkers of Stress and Listening Effort

There is currently no research available indicating how much cochlear implants may be able to impact one's degree of listening effort, although the anecdotal reports from clinical patients are noteworthy. Studies using measures of listening effort, such as pupillometry (e.g., Zekveld, Kramer, & Festen, 2010, 2011), heart rate variability (e.g., Dorman et al., 2012), or skin conductance (Mackersie & Cones, 2011), may provide assistance in determining the degree of benefit afforded by cochlear implantation for individuals with significant hearing loss. Furthermore, it is possible that measures of listening effort, objective or subjective, may also play a role in determining implant candidacy, particularly for patients who may be considered "borderline" candidates on the basis of audiometric testing.

Objective Estimates of Listening Effort

Pupillometry

There are a number of objective or physiologic correlates of listening effort. Pupils dilate in response to cognitive workload with peak dilation occurring approximately 1 to 2 s after demand onset. Measuring degree and latency of pupil dilation has been used for a number of years to gauge cognitive processing load for tasks including mathematics and academic testing complexity (Ahern & Beatty, 1979; Klinger et al., 2011) and memory recall (Kahneman & Beatty, 1966; Taylor, 1981; Granholm et al., 1996; Piquado, Isaacowitz, & Wingfield, 2010; Klinger et al., 2011). In recent years, pupil-dilation responses have been used as a metric of listening effort for individuals with and without hearing loss (Zekveld et al., 2010, 2011; Koelewijn, Zekveld, Festen, & Kramer, 2012). Audiology clinics that offer vestibular testing will likely already have video eye-tracking systems that can calculate pupil position for assessing oculomotor function. Pupillometry measures for gauging listening effort, however, will likely not be included in the clinical software because the triggering programs for synchronizing speech stimuli and the measurement of onset and peak dilation latency include specialized coding that is currently customized by individual research labs; thus, additional research is required to address its clinical applicability and efficacy for use in audiologic evaluation.

Heart Rate Variability

Heart rate variability (HRV) is a physiologic correlate of stress. HRV measurements reflect beat-to-beat variation in the natural heart rate, created by the actions of the sympathetic and parasympathetic branches of the autonomic nervous system. When under stress, activity of the sympathetic nervous system activity is higher thereby decreasing HRV. In less stressful conditions, there is greater activity of the parasympathetic nervous system thereby increasing HRV activity.

Dorman et al. (2012) showed significant decreases in HRV with increases in background noise levels as related to speech understanding for normal-hearing listeners; thus, it is possible that measures of HRV could be used to estimate the degree of auditory-related stress for individuals with hearing loss, and also potentially for supplementing the implant candidacy test battery. Although more research is clearly needed, the potential for clinical relevance is high. HRV measurement is rather simple and requires data from electrocardiogram (ECG) equipment that already exists in most major medical centers, although its applicability and ease of use in the audiology clinic is debatable without medically trained staff such as nurses or nursing assistants.

Skin Conductance

Skin conductance (also commonly referred to as galvanic skin response) is a measure reflecting the electrical conductance of the skin, which varies with moisture level. Skin moisture level is dependent on activity of the sweat glands, which are regulated by the sympathetic nervous system (primarily responsible for the body's "fight or flight" response); thus, skin conductance provides an indirect estimate of physiologic stress.

Mackersie and Cones (2011) evaluated the sensitivity of a number of physiologic markers of stress for gauging listening effort and task demand for individuals with normal hearing. Though they incorporated four physiologic measures of stress including heart rate, skin conductance, skin temperature, and electromyography, mean changes in skin conductance were found to be most sensitive to increasing task demand.

Skin conductance is currently measured best from the palm of the hand or the sole of the foot, because these areas have particularly dense populations of eccrine glands. Eccrine glands are involved in thermoregulation and are particularly sensitive to emotional triggers and mental demand. Measurement of skin conductance is most generally achieved with electrodes placed on the palm of the hand such as those employed during polygraph (lie-detector testing). Unlike ECG and oculomotor equipment as discussed previously for the measurement of HRV and pupil-dilation responses, skin-conductance measuring and analysis equipment may not be widely available in a medical center environment; thus, more research is necessary to address its clinical applicability and efficacy for use in audiologic evaluation.

Subjective Estimates of Listening Effort and Fatigue

Increased listening effort and auditory-related fatigue are known sequelae of hearing loss. Individuals with severe-to-profound hearing loss frequently report increased anxiety, stress, and mental fatigue in response to the communication demands in both their professional and social lives. These reports, however, are largely ignored in clinical practice despite the large social, emotional, and even financial impact.

Individuals with hearing loss have been shown to take significantly more sick leave due to stress-related complaints than individuals with normal hearing (Kramer, Kapteyn, & Houtgast, 2006; Nachtegaal, Festen, & Kramer, 2012). Individuals with hearing loss are also more likely to require longer recovery from work and work-related stress than individuals with normal hearing (Nachtegaal et al., 2009, 2012). Self-reported productivity at work is also negatively correlated with degree of hearing loss (Nachtegaal et al., 2012); thus, it makes sense to assess degree of auditory-related fatigue among individuals presenting for cochlear implant candidacy evaluation. It is possible that cochlear implantation may actually increase one's work productivity, although careful research is needed.

There are a number of questionnaires that were designed specifically to address subjective fatigue. These questionnaires, however, were not designed with auditory-related fatigue in mind. Rather, the majority of questionnaires were designed to assess fatigue as related to chronic health conditions such as cancer, autoimmune disease, and sleep disorders. It is currently unclear what applicability such instruments would have for individuals with auditory-related fatigue. There are researchers currently working in this area, and it is likely that the future will bring validated questionnaires designed to assess fatigue as related to hearing and hearing loss.

Children and Listening Effort

Auditory-based instruction is a vital part of a child's classroom experience (Figure 9–2). The effects of childhood hearing loss on listening effort and mental alertness can greatly impact learning and academic performance. A wealth of research suggests that a child's academic performance is greatly influenced by degree of mental alertness. Sleep has generally been attributed as the primary underlying factor affecting a child's mental alertness in the classroom (e.g., Eliasson, Eliasson, King, Gould, & Eliasson, 2002; Gozal, 1998; Perez-Chada et al., 2007; Ravid, Afek, Suraiya, Shahar, & Pillar, 2009). For children with hearing loss, however, sleep is not the only factor nor may it be the primary factor affecting academic performance.

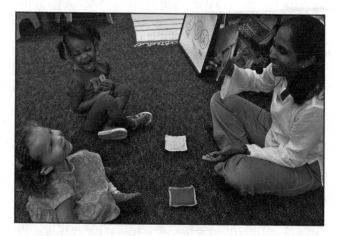

FIGURE 9–2. Auditory-based instruction, a vital part of a child's classroom experience, is shown.

Evidence exists that children with hearing loss expend greater listening effort than their peers with normal hearing (e.g., Bess et al., 1998; Hicks & Tharpe, 2002; Stelmachowicz, Lewis, Choi, & Hoover, 2007). This translates into greater fatigue, stress, and increased academic risk for children with hearing loss, even children with milder degrees of hearing loss than those presenting for cochlear implant candidacy (e.g., Bess et al., 1998; Tharpe, 2008). Children with hearing loss who do not meet the typical auditory profile for cochlear implant candidacy not only demonstrate speech-recognition benefits from cochlear implantation but may also experience decreased listening effort, fatigue, stress, and associated academic risk; thus, a clinical measure of listening effort may ultimately become a part of the pediatric battery for implant candidate assessment.

Older Adults and Listening Effort

Age is known to affect a host of cognitive processes including working memory (e.g., Salthouse, 1991, 1994; Span, Ridderinkhof, & van der Molen, 2004) and executive function (e.g., Span et al., 2004; Buckner, 2004; Mahoney, Verghese, Goldin, Lipton, & Holtzer, 2010); thus, it is not completely unexpected that older listeners have been shown to expend greater listening effort for speech recognition in noise than younger listeners (e.g., Anderson, Gosselin, & Gagne, 2011). This is thought to be related to the effect of age on global cognitive processing. In a similar vein, but from an auditory perspective, older individuals—even those with normal hearing—exhibit significantly poorer speech recognition in noise (Dubno, Horwitz, & Ahlstrom, 2002, 2003; Gifford, Bacon, & Williams, 2007; Smith, Pichora-Fuller, Wilson, & Macdonald, 2012). These age-related declines in speech recognition in noise are thought to be related to cognitive processing as well as age-related declines in auditory temporal processing (e.g., Strauss, Ashmead, Ohde & Grantham, 1998).

Relationships between age, cognitive processing, hearing loss, and speech recognition in noise are likely also entwined with the increased risk for incident dementia in older individuals (see section entitled "Dementia and Link with Hearing Loss"). As discussed in the previous section on children, it

is possible that clinical testing for degree of listening effort may ultimately assist adult implant candidate selection, especially for older adults who may be considered "borderline" candidates.

MULTISENSORY ASSESSMENT

Assessment of speech recognition both pre- and postoperatively involves the use of recorded speech stimuli presented in the sound field via audition only. Although this currently represents the standard of care assessment of speech recognition in clinical audiology, it is not a real-life assessment of communication abilities as we are rarely placed in situations during which all visual cues are absent. In fact, audiovisual integration is a significant part of communication for individuals who have access to multiple sensory modalities. For children with hearing loss, audiovisual integration is acquired via extensive early listening and communication experience.

Despite the audiovisual nature of speech communication, clinical practice has almost exclusively focused on speech testing in the auditory-only condition. The reason has primarily been to gauge listeners' abilities to understand speech in the most challenging conditions. Clinical measures of audiovisual speech recognition already exist for both children and adults. For pediatric multimodal speech-perception testing, there is the Children's Audio-Visual Enhancement Test (CAVET) (Tye-Murray & Geers, 2001) and the Audiovisual Feature Test (Tyler, Fryauf-Bertschy, & Kelsay, 1991). Both tests allow for auditory alone, visual alone, and audiovisual administration of stimuli. The CAVET is an open-set test of word recognition and includes three lists of 20 words. The Audiovisual Feature Test is a closed-set test that assesses recognition of consonant features.

Holt, Kirk, and Hay-McCutcheon (2011) have proposed more widespread use of audiovisual speech recognition for children. They reported on the development of an audiovisual version of the Lexical Neighborhood Sentence Test, which was adapted from the Lexical Sentence Test (Eisenberg, Martinez, Holowecky, & Pogorelsky, 2002). Holt and colleagues found that multimodal assessment of speech recognition was possible for children as young as 3 to 4 years for at least the auditory only and audiovisual conditions. Holt and colleagues further reported that there are plans to ultimately adapt the audiovisual Lexical Neighborhood Sentence Test for use in clinical practice. We can be certain that as the field evolves, the assessment of the whole child, including multimodal speech-perception abilities, will likely be integrated into the minimum pediatric speech-recognition test battery.

BILATERAL IMPLANT CANDIDACY: WHEN IS IT TIME TO CONSIDER A SECOND IMPLANT?

One of the most frequently asked questions of both clinicians and patients is, "When is the right time to consider a second implant?" Despite the wealth of published research on both bimodal and bilateral function, there are currently no well-defined guidelines that can direct clinicians who are assisting with or recommending such decisions. More specifically, there are no definitive reports highlighting audiometric profiles, configuration of hearing loss, levels of speech-perception performance, or levels of speech/language delay that can serve as preoperative indicators to determine whether an individual should pursue one or two implants.

Most patients being considered for cochlear implantation retain "bilateral" hearing in the sense that they either hear bimodally—with one cochlear implant and aided acoustic hearing in the nonimplanted ear—or receive two cochlear implants. At the time of chapter preparation, bilateral cochlear implantation was considered standard-of-care treatment for individuals with bilateral severe-to-profound sensorineural hearing loss for some of the largest of private health insurance companies in the United States including Aetna, Blue Cross Blue Shield, Cigna, Great West, Health Partners, Kaiser California, Medica, Priority Health, and TRICARE (though this list is not exhaustive). Furthermore, the William House Cochlear Implant Study Group (Balkany et al., 2008) and Papsin and Gordon (2008) have recognized bilateral cochlear implantation as accepted medical practice and stated that it should be considered standard-of-care treatment for severe-to-profound sensorineural hearing loss.

In order to make data-driven recommendations for a second implant, one must recognize that the efficacy of a particular intervention—in this case, a second cochlear implant—depends heavily on the tests used for its measurement. Such tests must be sensitive enough to gauge the relevant speech information provided by acoustic hearing in the case of bimodal hearing as well as the information provided by a second cochlear implant for bilateral implant recipients. This is much easier said than done.

For children acquiring spoken language via implant technology, there are an increasing number of reports indicating that bilateral cochlear implantation at a young age yields higher levels of speech perception (Lovett, Kitterick, Hewitt, & Summerfield, 2010; Wolfe et al., 2007), rapid language acquisition achieving age-appropriate norms at younger ages (Wie, 2010), binaural summation (Dorman et al., 2011; Buss, Pillsbury, Buchman, Pillsbury, Clark, Haynes, et al., 2008; Litovsky, Parkinson, Arcaroli, & Sammeth, 2006; Koch, Soli, Downing, & Osberger, 2010), equivalent head shadow across ears (Buss et al., 2008; Litovsky et al., 2006), binaural squelch (Buss et al., 2008; Eapen, Buss, Adunka, Pillsbury III, & Buchman, 2009), and improved localization abilities (Beijin, Snik, & Mylanus et al., 2007; Grieco-Calub & Litovsky, 2010; Godar & Litovsky, 2010; Lovett et al., 2010; van Deun et al., 2010).

For adults receiving a second cochlear implant, in addition to gains reported above for summation, squelch, and localization, there are large gains in health-related quality of life (QOL). On a dead/healthy scale of 0 to 1, where 0 represents death and 1 represents perfect health, adult implant recipients report significant QOL improvement from 0.69 with one implant to 0.81 with a second implant (Bichey & Miyamoto, 2008). In fact, the improvement reported with the second implant was almost equivalent to the improvement seen with the first implant, a concept that can be difficult to understand given the much larger *relative* improvement in speech recognition observed with the first implant. Perhaps even more surprising is that the health-related QOL improvement observed with the second implant represents a favorable cost utility—much more favorable, and hence much less expensive at face value, than even estrogen replacement therapy and medical treatment for hypertension (Bichey & Miyamoto, 2008); thus, one could conclude that recommending a second cochlear implant, when warranted, is truly a judicious use of health care funds.

It is those assessments which include the "whole patient" that are required in order to determine bilateral candidacy and efficacy of bilateral cochlear implantation, because the current clinical measures of speech perception, as well as speech and language outcomes, are not always sensitive to the effects of unilateral versus bilateral deafness. This is a fact that has been clearly outlined in the literature on minimal hearing loss (e.g., Bess & Tharpe, 1984, 1986; Oyler, Oyler, & Matkin, 1988; Tharpe & Bess, 1991; Tharpe, 2008). In other words, as long as a single implant provides significant communicative improvement, standardized measures of speech perception and speech/language development will likely not provide the information needed to determine candidacy or to assess postoperative effectiveness of bilateral implantation; thus, we will likely see more widespread clinical use of complex listening tasks, including multiple loudspeakers (Figure 9–3).

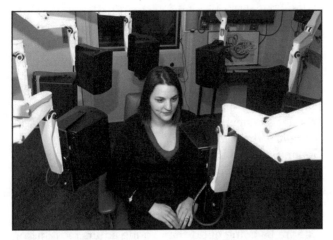

FIGURE 9–3. The R-SPACE (Revitronix, Braintree, VT) array of eight loudspeakers, which delivers proprietary restaurant-noise recordings from all speakers allowing for the assessment of speech recognition in a realistic listening environment (one in which noise originates from all around the listener rather than from a single loudspeaker placed in front, to the side, or to the back of the listener), is shown.

CONCLUSION

As clinicians we must strive to constantly challenge the status quo regarding standard of care and question whether our current tools are enough to identify patient concerns, to identify patients who may continue to struggle with communication in everyday listening environments, and to identify the *global* effectiveness of a particular treatment option. The latter concern, in particular, will certainly be considered by insurance and governmental agencies when proposing health care initiatives for cost containment. Though the field has made considerable strides in the management and assessment of patients with significant hearing loss, we still have much room for improvement.

Cochlear implants have been called the most successful neural prosthesis ever developed, and for this reason, cochlear implants may serve as a metaphorical blueprint in the development of other neural prosthetics such as those for the vestibular and visual systems (Wilson & Dorman, 2008). For clinicians who work with cochlear implant recipients, there is simply no other intervention in this field that yields such dramatic, life-altering outcomes. It is for this reason that we must continue to promote public awareness and eliminate barriers to this technology for those who may derive benefit. The future holds tremendous promise for adults and children with significant sensorineural hearing loss. With continued attention, research, assessment, and reassessment of our clinical management protocols, the possibilities will most certainly multiply.

REFERENCES

Ahern, S., & Beatty, J. (1979). Pupillary responses during information processing vary with Scholastic Aptitude Test scores. *Science, 205*(4412), 1289–1292.

Anderson Gosselin, P., & Gagne, J. P. (2011). Older adults expend more listening effort than young adults recognizing speech in noise. *Journal of Speech, Language, and Hearing Research, 54,* 944–958.

Balkany, T., Hodges, A., Telischi, F., Hoffman, R., Madell, J., Parisier, S., et al. (2008). William House Cochlear Implant Study Group: Position statement on bilateral cochlear implantation. *Otology & Neurotol, 29*(2),107–108.

Beijin, J. W., Snik, A. F., & Mylanus, E. A. (2007). Sound localization ability of young children with bilateral cochlear implants. *Otology & Neurotology, 8,* 479–485.

Bess, F. H., Dodd-Murphy, J., & Parker, R. A. (1998). Children with minimal sensorineural hearing loss: Prevalence, educational performance, and functional status. *Ear and Hearing, 19,* 339–354.

Bess, F. H., & Tharpe, A. M. (1984). Unilateral hearing impairment in children. *Pediatrics, 74,* 206–216.

Bess, F. H., & Tharpe, A. M. (1986). Case history data on unilaterally hearing-impaired children. *Ear and Hearing, 7,* 14–19.

Bichey, B. G., & Miyamoto, R. T. (2008). Outcomes in bilateral cochlear implantation. *Otolaryngology—Head and Neck Surgery, 138,* 655–661

Buckner, R. L. (2004). Memory and executive function in aging and AD: Multiple factors that cause decline and reserve factors that compensate. *Neuron, 44,* 195–208.

Buss, E., Pillsbury, H. C., Buchman, C. A., Pillsbury, C. H., Clark, M.S., Haynes, D. S., et al. (2008). Multicenter U.S. bilateral MED-EL cochlear implantation study: Speech perception over the first year of use. *Ear and Hearing, 29*(1), 20–32.

Dorman, M. F., Spahr, A. J., Gifford, R. H., Cook, S. J., Zhang, T., Loiselle, L., et al. (2012). Current research with cochlear implants at Arizona State University. *Journal of the American Academy of Audiology, 23,* 385–395.

Dorman, M. F., Yost, W. A., Wilson, B. A., & Gifford, R. H. (2011). Speech perception and sound localization with bilateral cochlear implants. *Seminars in Hearing, 32,* 73–89.

Downs, D. W. (1982). Effects of hearing aid use on speech discrimination and listening effort. *Journal of Speech and Hearing Disorders, 47,* 189–193.

Dubno, J. R., Horwitz, A. R., & Ahlstrom, J. B. (2002). Benefit of modulated maskers for speech recognition by younger and older adults with normal hearing. *Journal of the Acoustical Society of America, 111,* 2897–2907.

Dubno, J. R., Horwitz, A. R., & Ahlstrom, J. B. (2003). Recovery from prior stimulation: Masking of speech by interrupted noise for younger and older adults with normal hearing. *Journal of the Acoustical Society of America, 113,* 2084–2094.

Eapen, R. J., Buss, E., Adunka, M. C., Pillsbury, H. C. III, & Buchman, C. A. (2009). Hearing-in-noise benefits after bilateral simultaneous cochlear implanta-tion continue to improve 4 years after implantation. *Otology & Neurotology, 30,* 153–159

Eisenberg, L. S., Martinez, A. S., Holowecky, S. R., & Pogorelsky, S. (2002). Recognition of lexically controlled words and sentences by children with normal hearing and children with cochlear implants. *Ear and Hearing, 23*(5), 450–462.

Eliasson, A., Eliasson, A., King, J., Gould, B., & Eliasson, A. (2002). Association of sleep and academic performance. *Sleep and Breathing, 6,* 45–45.

Ferri, C. P., Prince, M., Brayne, C., Brodaty, H., Fratiglioni, L., Ganguli, M., et al. (2005). Global prevalence of dementia: A Delphi consensus study. *Lancet, 366,* 2112–2117.

Feuerstein, J. F. (1992). Monaural versus binaural hearing: Ease of listening, word recognition, and attentional effort. *Ear and Hearing, 13,* 80–86.

Folstein, M. F., Folstein, S. E., & McHugh, P. R. (1975). Mini-mental state. A practical method for grading the cognitive state of patients for the clinician. *Journal of Psychiatric Research, 12*(3), 189–198.

Fraser, S., Gagne, J. P., Alepins, M., & Dubois, P. (2010). Evaluating the effort expended to understand speech in noise using a dual-task paradigm: The effects of providing visual speech cues. *Journal of Speech, Language, and Hearing Research, 53,* 18–33.

Freitas, S., Simões, M. R., Alves, L., & Santana I. (2011). Montreal cognitive assessment: Validation study for mild cognitive impairment and Alzheimer disease. *Alzheimer Disease & Associated Disorders,* 2011 Dec 20. [Epub ahead of print].

Galvin, J. E., & Sadowsky, C. H. (2012). Practical guidelines for the recognition and diagnosis of dementia. *Journal of the American Board of Family Medicine, 25*(3), 367–382.

Gifford, R. H., Bacon, S. P., & Williams, E. J. (2007). An examination of speech recognition in a modulated background and of forward masking in younger and older listeners. *Journal of Speech, Language, and Hearing Research, 50,* 857–864.

Godar, S. P., & Litovsky, R. Y. (2010). Experience with bilateral cochlear implants improves sound localization acuity in children. *Otology & Neurotology, 31,* 1287–1292.

Gosselin, P. A., & Gagne, J. P. (2011). Older adults expend more listening effort than young adults recognizing audiovisual speech in noise. *Internatonal Journal of Audiology, 50,* 786–792.

Gozal, D. (1998). Sleep-disordered breathing and school performance in children. *Pediatrics, 102*(3 Pt 1), 606–620.

Granholm, E., Asarnow, R. F., Sarkin, A. J., & Dykes, K. L. (1996). Pupillary responses index cognitive resource limitations. *Psychophysiology, 33,* 457–461.

Grieco-Calub, T. M., & Litovsky, R. Y. (2010). Sound localization skills in children who use bilateral cochlear implants and in children with normal acoustic hearing. *Ear and Hearing, 31,* 645–656.

Hetu, R., Riverin, L., Lalande, N., Getty, L., & St-Cyr, C. (1988). Qualitative analysis of the handicap associated with occupational hearing loss. *British Journal of Audiology, 22*(4), 251–264.

Heydebrand, G., Hale, S., Potts, L., & Skinner, M. (2007). Cognitive predictors of improvements in adults' spoken word recognition six months after cochlear implant activation. *Audiology and Neurotology, 12,* 254–264.

Hicks, C. B., & Tharpe, A. M. (2002). Listening effort and fatigue in school-age children with and without hearing loss. *Journal of Speech, Language, and Hearing Research, 45,* 573–584.

Holt, R. F., Kirk, K. I., & Hay-McCutcheon, M. (2011). Assessing multimodal spoken word-in-sentence recognition in children with normal hearing and children with cochlear implants. *Journal of Speech, Language, and Hearing Research, 54*(2), 632–657.

Kahneman, D., & Beatty, J. (1966). Pupil diameter and load on memory. *Science, 154*(3756), 1583–1585.

Koch, D. B., Soli, S. D., Downing, M., & Osberger, M. J. (2010). Simultaneous bilateral cochlear implantation: Prospective study in adults. *Cochlear Implants International, 11*(2), 84–99

Kochkin, S. (2008). MarkeTrak VIII: 25-year trends in the hearing health market. *Hearing Review, 16,* 12–31.

Koelewijn, T., Zekveld, A. A., Festen, J. M., & Kramer, S. E. (2012). Pupil dilation uncovers extra listening effort in the presence of a single-talker masker. *Ear and Hearing, 33*(2), 291–300.

Kramer, S. E., Kapteyn, T. S., & Houtgast, T. (2006). Occupational performance: Comparing normally-hearing and hearing-impaired employees using the Amsterdam Checklist for Hearing and Work. *International Journal of Audiology, 45*(9), 503–512.

Kramer, S. E., Zekveld, A. A., & Houtgast, T. (2009). Measuring cognitive factors in speech comprehension: The value of using the text reception threshold test as a visual equivalent of the SRT test. *Scandinavian Journal of Psychology, 50,* 507–515.

Larner, A. J. (2012). Screening utility of the Montreal Cognitive Assessment (MoCA): In place of—or as well as—the MMSE? *International Psychogeriatrics, 24,* 391–396.

Lin, F. R. (2012). Hearing loss in older adults: Who's listening. *Journal of the American Medical Association, 307*(11), 1147–1148.

Lin, F. R., Metter, E. J., O'Brien, R. J., Resnick, S. M., Zonderman, A. B., & Ferrucci, L. (2011a). Hearing loss and incident dementia. *Archives of Neurology, 68*(2), 214–220.

Lin, F. R., Niparko, J. K., & Ferrucci, L. (2011b). Health care reform: Hearing loss prevalence in the United States. *Archives of Internal Medicine, 171,* 1851–1853.

Litovsky, R., Parkinson, A., Arcaroli, J., & Sammeth, C. (2006). Simultaneous bilateral cochlear implantation in adults: A multicenter clinical study. *Ear and Hearing, 27*(6), 714–731.

Lovett, R. E., Kitterick, P. T., Hewitt, C. E., & Summerfield, A. Q. (2010). Bilateral or unilateral cochlear implantation for deaf children: An observational study. *Archives of Disease in Childhood, 95,* 107–112.

Lyxell, B., Andersson, J., Arlinger, S., Bredberg, G., Harder, H., & Ronnberg, J. (1996). Verbal information-processing capabilities and cochlear implants: Implications for preoperative predictors of speech understanding. *Journal of Deaf Studies and Deaf Education, 1*(3), 190–201.

Mackersie, C. L., & Cones, H. (2011). Subjective and psychophysiological indexes of listening effort in a competing-talker task. *Journal of the American Academy of Audiology, 22,* 113–122.

Mahoney, J. R., Verghese, J., Goldin, Y., Lipton, R., & Holtzer, R. (2010). Alerting, orienting, and executive attention in older adults. *Journal of the International Neuropsychological Society, 16*(5), 877–889.

Moran, W. P., Zapka, J., Iverson, P. J., Zhao, Y., Wiley, M. K., Pride, P., et al. (2012). Aging Q3: An initiative to improve internal medicine residents' geriatrics knowledge, skills, and clinical performance. *Academic Medicine, 87*(5), 635–642.

Nachtegaal, J., Festen, J. M., & Kramer, S. E. (2012). Hearing ability in working life and its relationship with sick leave and self-reported work productivity. *Ear and Hearing, 33*(1), 94–103.

Nachtegaal, J., Kuik, D. J., Anema, J. R., Goverts, S. T., Festen, J. M., & Kramer, S. E. (2009). Hearing status, need for recovery after work, and psychosocial work characteristics: Results from an Internet-based national survey on hearing. *International Journal of Audiology, 48*(10), 684–691.

Nasreddine, Z., Phillips, N. A., & BeaLdirian, V. (2005). The Montreal Cognitive Assessment, MoCA: A brief screening tool for Mild Cognitive Impairment. *Journal of the American Geriatric Society, 53,* 695–699.

Nazem, S., Siderowf, A. D., Duda, J. E., Have, T. T., Colcher, A., Horn, S. S., Moberg, P. J., Wilkinson, J. R., Hurtig, H. I., Stern, M. B., & Weintraub, D. (2009). Montreal cognitive assessment performance in patients with Parkinson's disease with "normal" global cognition according to mini-mental state examination score. *Journal American Geriatric Society, 57,* 304–308.

Oyler, R. F., Oyler, A. L., & Matkin, N. D. (1988). Unilateral hearing loss: Demographics and educational impact. *Language, Speech, and Hearing Services in Schools, 19,* 201–210.

Papsin, B. C., & Gordon, K. A. (2008). Bilateral cochlear implants should be the standard for children with bilateral sensorineural deafness. *Current Opinion in Otolaryngology & Head and Neck Surgery, 16,* 69–74.

Peelle, J. E., Troiani, V., Grossman, M., & Wingfield, A. (2011). Hearing loss in older adults affects neural systems supporting speech comprehension. *Journal of Neuroscience, 31*(35), 12638–12643.

Perez-Chada, D., Perez-Lloret, S., Videla, A. J., Cardinali, D., Bergna, M. A., et al. (2007). Sleep disordered breathing and daytime sleepiness are associated with poor academic performance in teenagers. A study using the Pediatric Daytime Sleepiness Scale (PDSS). *Sleep, 30,* 1698–1703.

Pichora-Fuller, M. K. (2007). Audition and cognition: What audiologists need to know about listening. In C. Palmer & R. Seewald (Eds.), *Hearing care for adults* (pp. 71–85). Stafa, Switzerland: Phonak.

Piquado, T., Isaacowitz, D., & Wingfield, A. (2010). Pupillometry as a measure of cognitive effort in younger and older adults. *Psychophysiology, 47,* 560–569.

Pisoni, D. B. (2000). Cognitive factors and cochlear implants: Some thoughts on perception, learning and memory in speech perception. *Ear and Hearing, 21,* 70–78.

Prince, M., & Jackson, J. (Eds.). (2009). *Alzheimer's disease international.* World Alzheimer Report 2009.

Ravid, S., Afek, I., Suraiya, S., Shahar, E., & Pillar, G. (2009). Kindergarten children's failure to qualify for first grade could result from sleep disturbances. *Journal of Childhood Neurology, 24,* 816–822.

Ronnberg, J., Rudner, M., Foo, C., et al. (2008). Cognition counts: A working memory system for ease of language understanding. *International Journal of Audiology, 47,* S99–S105.

Rossi-Katz, J., & Arehart, K. H. (2011). Survey of audiologic service provision to older adults with cochlear implants. *American Journal of Audiology, 20*(2), 84–89.

Salthouse, T. A. (1991). Mediation of adult age difference in cognitive by reductions in working memory and speed of processing. *Psychological Science, 2,* 179–183.

Salthouse, T. A. (1994). The aging of working memory. *Neuropsychology, 8,* 535–543.

Shinn-Cunningham, B. G., & Best, V. (2008). Selective attention in normal and impaired hearing. *Trends in Amplification, 12*(4), 283–299

Simmons, B. B., Hartmann, B., & Dejoseph, D. (2011). Evaluation of suspected dementia. *American Family Physician, 84*(8), 895–902.

Smith, S. L., Pichora-Fuller, M. K., Wilson, R. H., & Macdonald, E. N. (2012). Word recognition for temporally and spectrally distorted materials: The effects of age and hearing loss. *Ear and Hearing, 33*(3), 349–366.

Span, M. M., Ridderinkhof, K. R., & van der Molen, M. W. (2004). Age-related changes in the efficiency of cognitive processing across the life span. *Acta Psychologica (Amsterdam), 117*(2), 155–183.

Stelmachowicz, P. G., Lewis, D. E., Choi, S., & Hoover, B. (2007). The effect of stimulus bandwidth on auditory skills in normal-hearing and hearing-impaired children. *Ear and Hearing, 28*(4), 483–494.

Steven, R. A., Green, K. M., Broomfield, S. J., Henderson, L. A., Ramsden, R. T., & Bruce, I. A. (2011). Cochlear implantation in children with cerebral palsy. *International Journal of Pediatric Otorhinolaryngology, 75*(11), 1427–1430.

Strouse, A., Ashmead, D. H., Ohde, R. N., & Grantham, D. W. (1998). Temporal processing in the aging auditory system. *Journal of the Acoustical Society of America, 104,* 2385–2399.

Tay, T., Wang, J. J., Kifley, A., Lindley, R., Newall, P., & Mitchel, P. (2006). Sensory and cognitive association in older persons: Findings from an older Australian population. *Gerontology, 52*(6), 386–394.

Taylor, J. S. (1981). Pupillary response to auditory versus visual mental loading: A pilot study using super 8-mm photography. *Perceptual and Motor Skills, 52*(2), 425–426.

Tharpe, A. M. (2008). Unilateral and mild bilateral hearing loss in children: Past and current perspectives. *Trends in Amplification, 12,* 7–15.

Tharpe, A. M., & Bess, F. H. (1991). Identification and management of children with minimal hearing loss. *International Journal of Pediatric Otorhinolaryngology, 21,* 41–50.

Tye-Murray, N., & Geers, A. (2001). *Children's audiovisual enhancement test.* St. Louis, MO: Central Institute for the Deaf.

Tyler, R. S., Fryauf-Bertschy, H., & Kelsay, D. (1991). *Audiovisual feature test for young children.* Iowa City, IA: University of Iowa.

United Nations. (2010). *World population prospects: The 2010 revision.* Retrieved from http://esa.un.org/unpd/wpp

U.S. Census. (2010). Retrieved June 29, 2012, from http://www.census.gov

Van Deun, L., van Wieringer, A., Scherf, F., Doggouj, N., Desloovere, C., Offeciers, F. E., et al. (2010). Earlier intervention leads to better sound localization in children with bilateral cochlear implants. *Audiology and Neurotology, 15,* 7–17.

Wie, O. B. (2010). Language development in children after receiving bilateral cochlear implants between 5 and 18 months. *International Journal of Pediatric Otorhinolaryngology, 74,* 1258–1266.

Wilson, B. A., & Dorman, M. F. (2008). Interfacing sensors with the nervous system: Lessons from the development and success of the cochlear implant. *IEEE Sensors Journal, 8,* 131–147.

Wingfield, A., Tun, P. A., & McCoy, S. L. (2005). Hearing loss in older adulthood: What it is and how it interacts with cognitive performance. *Current Directions in Psychological Science, 14*(3), 144–148.

Wolfe, J., Baker, S., Caraway, T., Kasulis, H., Mears, A., Smith, J., et al. (2007). 1-year postactivation results for sequentially implanted bilateral cochlear implant users. *Otology & Neurotology, 28,* 589–596.

United Nations, Department of Economic and Social Affairs, Population Division. (2011). *World population prospects: The 2010 revision, volume II: Demographic profiles.* ST/ESA/SER.A/317.

World Health Organization and U.S. National Institute of Aging (2011). *Global health and aging.* NIH Publication No. 11–7737.

Zekveld, A. A., George, E. L. J., Kramer, S. E., Goverts, S. T., Houtgast, T. (2007). The development of the text reception threshold test: A visual analogue of the speech reception threshold test. *Journal of Speech, Language, and Hearing Research, 50,* 576–584.

Zekveld, A. A., Kramer, S. E., & Festen, J. M. (2010). Pupil response as an indication of effortful listening: The influence of sentence intelligibility. *Ear and Hearing, 31,* 480–490.

Zekveld, A. A., Kramer, S. E., & Festen, J. M. (2011). Cognitive load during speech perception in noise: The influence of age, hearing loss, and cognition on the pupil response. *Ear and Hearing, 32*(4), 498–510.

Index